Orthopaedic Office and Emergency Procedures

Orthopaedic Office and Emergency Procedures

C. MAX HOSHINO, MD

Assistant Chief
Orthopaedic Trauma Surgery
Harbor-UCLA Medical Center
Torrance, California

JOHN V. TIBERI III, MD

South Bay Orthopaedic Specialists
Medical Center
Torrance, California

THOMAS G. HARRIS, MD

Chief
Foot and Ankle Surgery
Harbor-UCLA Medical Center
Torrance, California
Director
Foot and Ankle Surgery
Congress Medical Associates
Pasadena, California

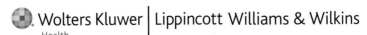

Wolters Kluwer | Lippincott Williams & Wilkins
Health
Philadelphia · Baltimore · New York · London
Buenos Aires · Hong Kong · Sydney · Tokyo

Acquisitions Editor: Brian Brown
Product Manager: Dave Murphy
Production Project Manager: Bridgett Dougherty
Director of Marketing Medical Practice: Lisa Zoks
Design Coordinator: Stephen Druding
Production Services: S4Carlisle Publishing Services

Printed in China

Library of Congress Cataloging-in-Publication Data

ISBN-13: 978-1-4511-4370-6

Cataloging-in-Publication data available on request from the Publisher.

To purchase additional copies of this book, call our customer service department at (800) 638-3030 or fax orders to (301) 223-2320. International customers should call (301) 223-2300.

Visit Lippincott Williams & Wilkins on the Internet: at LWW.com. Lippincott Williams & Wilkins customer service representatives are available from 8:30 am to 6:00 pm, EST.

10 9 8 7 6 5 4 3 2 1

RRS1309

To my loving wife for her unwavering support every step of the way.
To my parents for always supporting me in achieving my goals.

—CMH

To my mentors and colleagues, whose inspiration contributed to the
conception of this book.
To my wife Lindsay and my family for their unconditional support
throughout my life.
And to the surgeons, physicians, residents, and students that I hope will
benefit from this book in the future.

—JVT

To our two newest sources of inspiration: Cole and Kirra.
To my parents Tom and Sue and brother Brian, who taught me the power
of family and love.
To my mentor Dr. Ron Smith, who taught me the value of both preparation
and diligence.
And mostly for my loving, amazing wife and constant inspiration, Tiffany,
who teaches me every day.
Thank you all so very much.

—TGH

Preface

The goal of this book is to aid medical students, allied health professionals, and physicians in understanding and performing common musculoskeletal procedures. As medical students and junior residents, we frequently referred to handbooks before treating patients. For instance, when treating a patient with a distal radius fracture, we would use a handbook to review the relevant anatomy, radiographic parameters, and indications for surgery. However, often the handbook would advise a "closed reduction and immobilization," with the important technical details required to perform the procedure absent. As we quickly found out, no book existed that detailed the steps that are required to properly reduce and immobilize common injuries that we were encountering. Instead, information regarding cast and splint application, local anesthesia administration, and reduction techniques was passed down to us by our supervising residents, fellows, and attending physicians.

We began to document the steps required for common procedures, so as we progressed, through our training, to become the supervising physicians, we would have a consistent foundation of information. *Orthopaedic Office and Emergency Procedures* is the result of these notes. This text provides the clinician with a step-by-step guide to performing the most common musculoskeletal procedures. We detail the steps required to properly treat both patients with acute injuries in the emergency room and degenerative conditions in the office. Each procedure is described from start to finish, with recommended anesthesia techniques, patient positioning, steps required to complete each task, and proper immobilization (if required). Additionally, practical tips and tricks that we have learned by treating large number of patients are described.

Since the book was created from our clinical experience, it represents our bias in treating these conditions. In many cases, there are multiple techniques that can be implemented with good clinical results. While we did attempt to provide alternative approachs for many procedures, the reader should use their clinical judgment to determine the best treatment for an individual patient. We hope that readers find this a useful guide to aid them in the treatment of their patients.

C. Max Hoshino, MD
John V. Tiberi, MD
Thomas G. Harris, MD

Contents

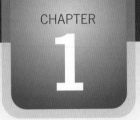

1

Basics of Splint and Cast Application

GENERAL PRINCIPLES

Splint versus Cast

In many situations, there are both splinting and casting options that will be effective in immobilizing the desired portion of the limb. A splint is not circumferential and, thus, accommodates swelling. In the acute setting, a splint is typically recommended because the eventual amount of soft tissue swelling is unpredictable. Because a cast is circumferential, it is stronger and more rigid. It offers increased stability and the ability to mold in all planes, which makes it more effective in holding reductions of unstable fractures. In the setting of an acute injury, a cast may be applied and is either uni- or bivalved to accommodate soft tissue swelling; however, it will still not be as soft tissue friendly as a splint (Fig. 1-1). Cast saws are designed to limit skin injury, but mechanical and thermal injury can still occur with improper usage. To prevent mechanical injury, place your index finger on the cast as a guard against plunging the saw too deep. To prevent thermal injury do not plow continuously through the cast. Rather, cut a small section of cast the width of the blade then disengage the saw completely prior to cutting the next section.

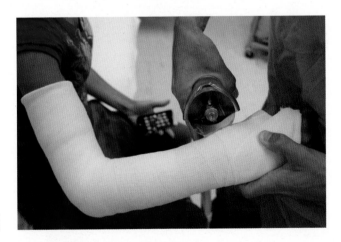

FIGURE
1-1

Splint and Cast Thickness

The ideal splint or cast is thick enough to have the strength to be rigid and to withstand associated forces while not being unnecessarily heavy or placing the patient at risk for thermal injury during the setting process. For plaster splints, we typically use 8 to 12 layers for the upper extremity and 12 to 15 layers for the lower extremity. Fiberglass is stronger than plaster, so fewer layers (typically 1/2 to 2/3 of the number of plaster layers) can be used.

Splint and Cast Padding

Cast padding is available in a variety of types and sizes; however, the principles are the same. Padding can be applied in a circumferential manner to the limb or as sheets corresponding to the predetermined length of the splint. Typically, cast padding cannot be applied excessively tight because it is designed to tear beyond an unsafe pressure. A minimum of two layers should be applied in any situation with more padding being required for fragile soft tissue and skin, for thicker casts or splints, around bony prominences, and at the anticipated site for a mold. In the setting of a cast, the padding is typically rolled circumferentially around the limb; while splinting, it may be applied in this manner or as longitudinal sheets along the inside of the splint. Regardless of the method, the padding should be applied slightly farther than the anticipated plaster or fiberglass to ensure adequate protection for the patient. If a cast or splint is to be applied over a wound, ensure that sufficient gauze or other dressing material is applied to absorb blood. When blood that is absorbed by the padding dries it becomes rigid, essentially creating a "blood cast" that will not allow swelling. To prevent this use the longitudinal sheet padding technique whenever bleeding is expected (e.g. open fractures, postoperative splint) (Figs. 1-2 and 1-3).

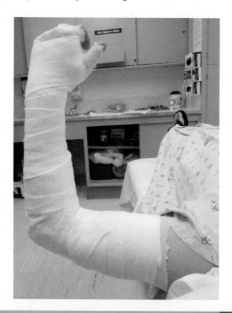

FIGURE
1-2

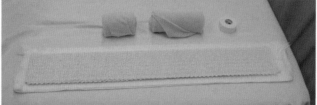

FIGURE
1-3

Splint Width

Splinting material comes in a variety of different widths, but is most frequently stocked in 4, 5, and 6 inch widths. The practitioner must chose the correct width based on the size of the patient and the area of the body. If the splint is too narrow, then the strength of the splint will be insufficient to stabilize the limb. On the other hand, an excessively wide splint will be circumferential, reducing the ability of the splint to accommodate swelling. In general, most splints distal to the elbow are made with 4 inch plaster. For the elbow and humerus 5 inch plaster is often used. For the lower extremity 5 or 6 inch plaster is used. However, the width of the splinting material should be adapted for larger (obese or muscular) or smaller (frail or pediatric) patients.

Temperature Concerns

An exothermic reaction occurs when water is added to splinting material, therefore heat is released in close proximity to the patient's skin. This results in the potential for burns. The amount of heat that reaches the skin is proportional to the plaster thickness, amount of padding, and water temperature. Since the amount of heat is proportional to the plaster thickness, the thinnest splint that is clinically effective should be used. It is very important to accurately measure the length of the splint, because the common practice of folding over the end of the splint to shorten an incorrectly measured splint doubles the plaster thickness at the end. This causes the end of splint to reach high temperatures, possibly resulting in thermal injury. With warmer water, plaster and fiberglass will set in a shorter amount of time but also reach higher temperatures. It is critical to understand that the temperature inside of the cast or splint (closer to the patient) is greater and dissipates slower than the temperature outside. Using cold water is always safest, and we do not recommend using water that is warmer than the ambient room temperature. Finally, the limb should not be placed on a pillow while the splint hardens. Pillows, especially the plastic type that are frequently used in hospitals, will not allow for dissipation of heat resulting in high temperatures near the patient's skin. The limb must be held as the splint or cast hardens to allow for heat dissipation.

Wrapping Cast Material around Joints

When a joint is immobilized in a position of some flexion, there will be a concave and convex side. The tendency is to place an excessive amount of casting material on the concave side while leaving the convex side too thin. To avoid this error, consider placing sheets of cut material or "fan-folding" along the convex side (Figs. 1-4 through 1-6).

Splint Overwrapping Material

One of the advantages of a splint over a cast is that the noncircumferential nature of the splint accommodates swelling of the soft tissue. With this concept in mind, select an appropriate material to overwrap the splint. Commonly used materials are bias (stockinette cut with a bias to create a single layer) and elastic bandages. Bias is preferred to elastic bandages for 3 reasons. Bias allows for the release of heat reducing the likelihood of thermal injury, and moisture reducing skin maceration and splint/cast weight as the plaster dries. Additionally, bias more uniformly distributes compression as the splint is wrapped. A gauze roll is a poor choice because it does not expand and is circumferentially restrictive. Similarly, tape should be applied in a nonrestricting manner.

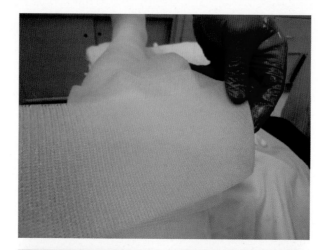

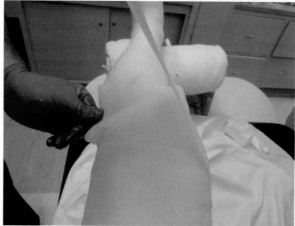

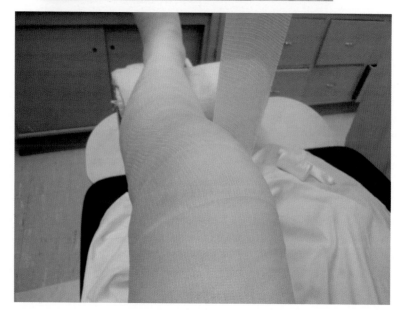

Molding

Molding of a cast or a splint is essential. It is important in maintaining a reduction by neutralizing deforming forces and in preventing movement or slipping through contours to the corresponding limb. Molds can also be dangerous to the soft tissues if not performed correctly. A proper mold occurs over broad surfaces to prevent areas of high pressure. Fingertips should never be used. Instead, use the palm of the hand or the thenar eminence. Additional cast padding can be used in areas of anticipated molds; however, it should be recognized that while additional layers of padding offer increased protection, excessive padding can increase the likelihood that the reduction will be lost once the swelling subsides. Plaster or fiberglass can be used. Plaster takes more time to set, allowing additional time for cast or splint application and molding; however, with an experienced assistant, fiberglass may be easier to mold since the position is required to be held for a shorter duration of time.

Wedging Casts

Wedging a cast is performed to correct fracture malalignment during the early stages of non-operative treatment. The first step is to determine the plane of malalignment by reviewing the patient's radiographs. For example, a varus malalignment of a tibia fracture will be seen on the AP radiograph. The apex of the deformity is then located to determine the location of the cast wedge. Either an opening wedge or a closing wedge can be performed. In the previous example of a varus malalignment of the tibia, an opening wedge can be performed on the medial side or a closing wedge on the lateral side to correct the deformity. We usually prefer an opening wedge to a closing wedge because the latter can result in skin becoming incarcerated in the closed wedge or bunching of cast padding. To perform an opening wedge, the cast is sectioned for three quarters of its circumference at the apex of the deformity. There are a number of techniques to determine the size of the wedge. We draw a longitudinal line representing the long axis of the bone on each side of the fracture. Cast wedges are then placed until this line becomes straight. A radiograph is then taken to confirm acceptable alignment. The opening is then padded, and the cast is rewrapped with fiberglass or plaster.

THE UPPER EXTREMITY

Coaptation Splint

Indication

The application of a coaptation splint is most commonly performed in the setting of a fracture of the humerus. It is the easiest and most effective way to immobilize the arm in an acute setting.

Description of Procedure

- Use the patient's unaffected arm to approximate the length of the splint. The appropriate length extends from the axilla along the medial aspect of the arm, around the elbow, and over the shoulder to at least the level of the acromioclavicular joint, preferably slightly longer (Fig. 1-7).
- Apply sufficient cast padding (see "Cast Padding" section discussed previously).
- With the elbow bent to 90°, apply the splint as high as possible in the axilla without causing discomfort or compression of the sensitive soft tissue or neurovascular structures in

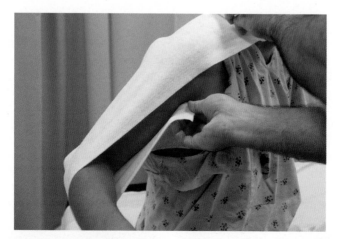

FIGURE
1-7

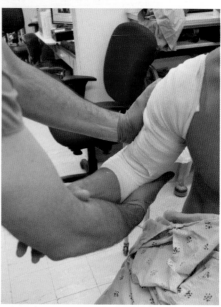

FIGURE
1-8

FIGURE
1-9

this area. The splint courses along the medial aspect of the arm, around the elbow, up the lateral aspect of the arm, and over the shoulder toward the neck (Fig. 1-8).

■ Wrap the splint with bias, and apply the desired mold (Fig. 1-9).

Long Arm Posterior Splint

Indication

A long arm splint is most commonly used for temporary treatment of injuries around or involving the elbow. It is effective in immobilizing the wrist, forearm, elbow, and a portion of the humerus.

Description of Procedure

- Use the patient's unaffected arm to approximate the length of the splint. The appropriate length extends along the posterior aspect of the arm and forearm beginning just distal to the shoulder and ending at the metacarpal heads. The forearm is routinely placed in neutral rotation; however, it may also be placed in supination or pronation (Fig. 1-10).
- Apply sufficient cast padding (see "Cast Padding" section discussed previously).
- With the elbow bent to 90° and the forearm supinated, apply the splint along the posterior aspect of the arm, elbow, wrist, and hand, ending at the metacarpal heads.
- Wrap the splint with bias (Fig. 1-11).

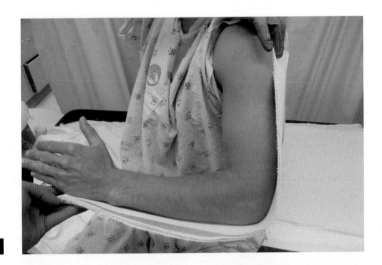

FIGURE
1-10

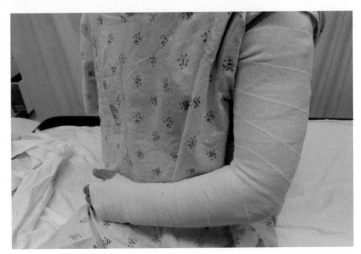

FIGURE
1-11

Long Arm Cast

Indication

A long arm cast is similar to a long arm posterior splint in that it is effective in immobilizing the wrist, forearm, elbow, and a portion of the humerus. Because a cast is circumferential, it is more amenable to molding but may not be appropriate in the acute setting with significant soft tissue edema.

Description of Procedure

- Apply sufficient cast padding (see "Cast Padding" section discussed previously) (Fig. 1-12).
- Begin wrapping plaster or fiberglass at the hand and wrist and continue proximally to the upper arm (Fig. 1-13).
- Maintenance of consistent wrist, forearm, and elbow position during the application of the cast is essential, as manipulation of these joints after the plaster or fiberglass has been applied will create wrinkles or distortion of the casting material that can become pressure points, placing the patient at risk for ulceration.
- While the plaster or fiberglass is still pliable, apply and hold the desired mold.

Tips and Other Considerations

- A long arm cast can be applied in two stages, if desired. First, apply a short arm cast (see "Short Arm Cast"), leaving some uncovered cast padding at the proximal portion of the cast. After the short arm cast has been appropriately molded and has hardened, extend the cast padding above the elbow; do not wrap cast padding over the plaster or fiberglass on the

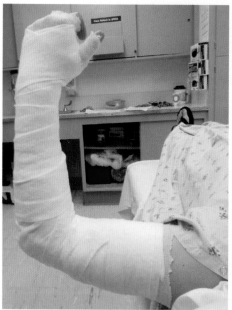

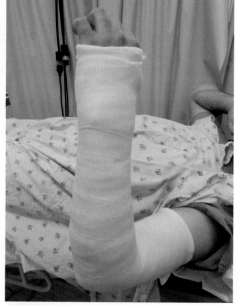

FIGURE
1-12

FIGURE
1-13

forearm that has already hardened (this will prevent the extended casting material from adhering to the short arm cast). Next, extend the casting material above the elbow. In order to avoid a weak transition point, begin wrapping cast material far distal to the transition point.

Hanging Arm Cast

Indication

The hanging arm cast is occasionally used for definitive nonoperative treatment of humerus shaft fractures with shortening.

Description of Procedure

▪ Apply a long arm cast with the elbow at 90° and the forearm in neutral rotation (see "Long Arm Cast"). The cast must extend 2 cm or more above the fracture site.

▪ Drop a plumb line from the midline of the neck to the cast and secure a ring to the cast at this point.

▪ To correct varus angulation, place the ring more dorsally (away from the body). To correct valgus angulation, place the ring more volarly (toward the body) (Fig. 1-14).

▪ To correct apex anterior angulation, place the ring more distally. To correct apex posterior angulation, place the ring more proximally (Fig. 1-14).

▪ Then suspend the cast by wrapping a strap through the ring and around the shoulders.

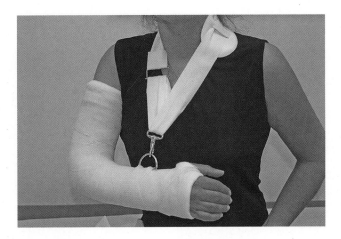

FIGURE
1-14

Single and Double Sugar-Tong Splint

Indication

Both single and double sugar-tong splints are commonly used for temporary treatment of injuries around or involving the arm and wrist. They are effective in immobilizing the wrist, forearm, and elbow. While a double sugar-tong splint is considerably heavier, there may be less of a tendency to slip off the elbow.

Description of Procedure

- Use the patient's unaffected arm to approximate the length of the splint. With the elbow bent 90° and the forearm in neutral rotation, the lower, or "single," portion should extend from just proximal to the metacarpal heads at the first palmar crease (to allow for full flexion of the MCP joints) on the palmar surface of the hand, along the volar surface of the forearm, around the elbow, and dorsally along the forearm and hand to the distal most aspect of the metacarpal heads.
- Apply sufficient cast padding (see "Cast Padding" section discussed previously).
- Apply the splint as described above, and wrap with bias (Figs. 1-15 through 1-17).
- After the plaster or fiberglass has set, the upper portion can be applied if desired. The upper, or "double," portion extends medially from the axilla, around the elbow, and laterally as proximal as desired (but at least as proximal as its medial extent).
- Apply sufficient cast padding (see "Cast Padding" section discussed previously) if not already done.
- Apply the splint as described above, and wrap with bias (Figs. 1-18 and 1-19).
- While the plaster or fiberglass is still pliable, apply and hold the desired mold.

Tips and Other Considerations

- It is typically easier to apply cast padding in sheets along the inner surface of the splinting material, as opposed to circumferentially around the upper extremity.
- The upper, or "double," portion of the splint can be extended into a coaptation splint if shoulder immobilization is necessary.
- With both a single and double sugar-tong splint, a sling will help immobilize the elbow and prevent slipping or breakdown of the splint.

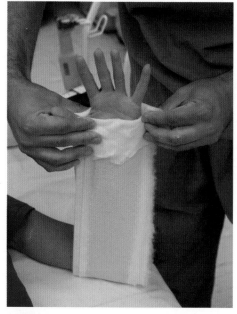

FIGURE
1-15

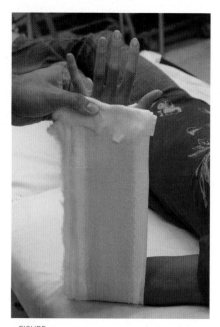

FIGURE
1-16

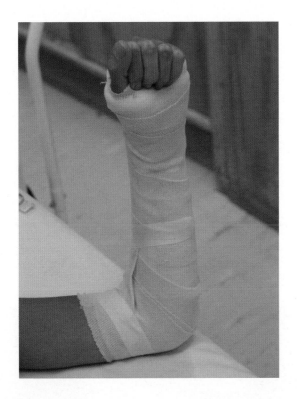

FIGURE
1-17

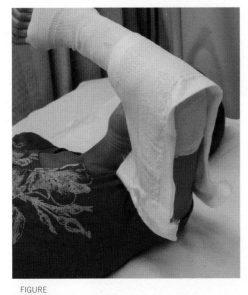

FIGURE
1-18

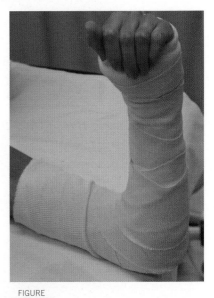

FIGURE
1-19

Volar Wrist Splint

Indication

A volar wrist splint is most commonly used for temporary treatment of injuries around or involving the wrist. It is effective in immobilizing volar–dorsal and radial–ulnar motion of the wrist and a portion of the forearm. Complete rotational control is not achieved because the proximal radioulnar joint is not immobilized.

Description of Procedure

- Use the patient's unaffected arm to approximate the length of the splint. The appropriate length extends just proximal to the metacarpal heads at the first palmar crease (to allow for full flexion of the MCP joints) on the palmar surface of the hand and along the volar surface of the forearm as proximal as possible but distal enough to avoid significant impingement of the splint when the elbow is flexed.
- Apply sufficient cast padding (see "Cast Padding" section discussed previously).
- Apply the plaster or fiberglass in the position described above (Fig. 1-20).
- Wrap with bias (Fig. 1-21).

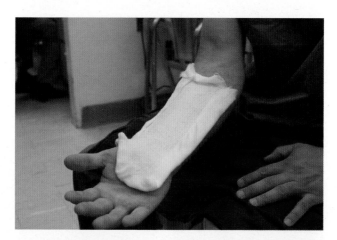

FIGURE
1-20

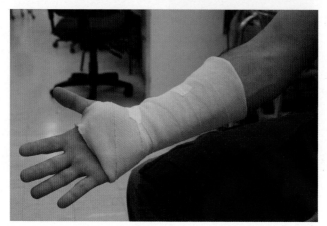

FIGURE
1-21

Tips and Other Considerations

▪ The volar wrist splint is most indicated in the treatment of soft tissue injuries or extremely stable bony injuries. It is far inferior to both casts and sugar-tong splints in maintaining reductions because it cannot be effectively molded.

Dorsal Wrist Splint

Indication

A dorsal wrist splint is most commonly used for temporary treatment of injuries around or involving the wrist. It is effective in immobilizing volar–dorsal and radial–ulnar motion of the wrist and a portion of the forearm. Complete rotational control is not achieved because the proximal radioulnar joint is not immobilized.

Description of Procedure

▪ Use the patient's unaffected arm to approximate the length of the splint. The appropriate length extends from the metacarpal heads along the dorsal surface of the forearm just distal to the elbow.
▪ Apply sufficient cast padding (see "Cast Padding" section discussed previously).
▪ Apply the plaster or fiberglass in the position described above (Fig. 1-22).
▪ Wrap with bias (Fig. 1-23).

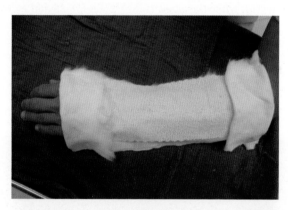

FIGURE
1-22

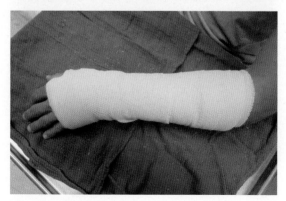

FIGURE
1-23

Tips and Other Considerations

■ Similar to the volar wrist splint, the dorsal wrist splint is most indicated in the treatment of soft tissue injuries or extremely stable bony injuries. It is far inferior to both casts and sugar-tong splints in maintaining reductions because it cannot be effectively molded.

Short Arm Cast

Indication

A short arm cast is similar to volar and dorsal wrist splints in that it is effective in immobilizing volar–dorsal and radial–ulnar motion of the wrist and a portion of the forearm without achieving complete rotational control because the proximal radioulnar joint is not immobilized. Because a cast is circumferential, it is more amenable to molding but may not be appropriate in the acute setting with significant soft tissue edema.

Description of Procedure

■ Apply sufficient cast padding (see "Cast Padding" section discussed previously) (Fig. 1-24).
■ Begin wrapping plaster or fiberglass at the hand and wrist and continue proximally to the upper forearm.
■ Ensure that the cast does not extend distally past the first palmar crease in order to allow MCP joint flexion. Similarly, extend as far proximal as possible but distal enough to avoid impingement of the cast while the elbow is flexed (Figs. 1-25 and 1-26).
■ Maintenance of consistent wrist and forearm position during the application of the cast is essential, as manipulation of these joints after the plaster or fiberglass has been applied will create wrinkles or distortion of the casting material that can become pressure points, placing the patient at risk for ulceration.
■ While the plaster or fiberglass is still pliable, apply and hold the desired mold.

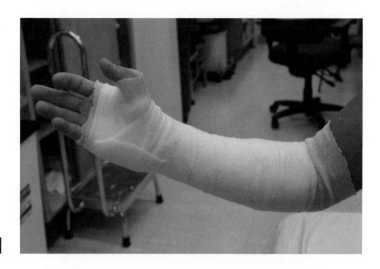

FIGURE
1-24

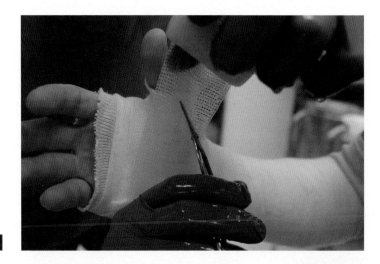

FIGURE
1-25

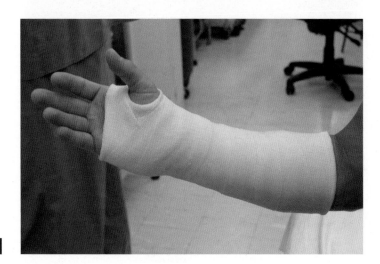

FIGURE
1-26

Ulnar Gutter Splint

Indication

An ulnar gutter splint is typically used for immobilization of the MCP, PIP, and DIP joints. Although it can be extended radially to treat the middle and index finger, it is most effective and most commonly used to treat metacarpal and proximal phalanx fractures of the small and ring fingers. Additionally, it is effective in immobilizing volar–dorsal and radial–ulnar motion of the wrist and a portion of the forearm. Complete rotational control is not achieved because the proximal radioulnar joint is not immobilized.

Description of Procedure

▪ Use the patient's unaffected arm to approximate the length of the splint. The appropriate length extends from the fingertips along the ulnar boarder of the hand, wrist, and forearm to just distal to the elbow.

▪ Apply sufficient cast padding (see "Cast Padding" section discussed previously).

▪ With the DIPs, PIPs, MCPs in extension and the wrist in neutral flexion/extension, apply the splinting material (Fig. 1-27).

▪ Wrap with bias.

▪ Maintain extension at the DIPs and PIPs while flexing the MCPs to 90° (Fig. 1-28).

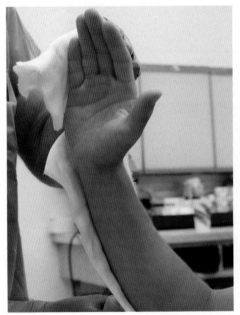

FIGURE
1-27

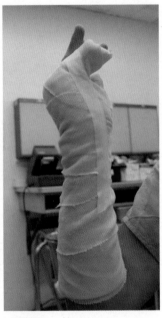

FIGURE
1-28

Tips and Other Considerations

▪ It is typically easier to apply cast padding in sheets along the inner surface of the splinting material, as opposed to circumferentially around the upper extremity.

▪ A common error with the ulnar gutter splint is failure to achieve MCP flexion due to excessive accumulation of splinting and padding material at the volar aspect of the MCP joint during splint application when the MCPs are flexed to 90°. To avoid this malposition, after the splint and padding have been measured but before it has been applied, mark the position that will correspond to the MCP joints. Using bandage scissors, remove some of the splinting and padding material from this location. Proceed with the application of the splint (Fig. 1-29).

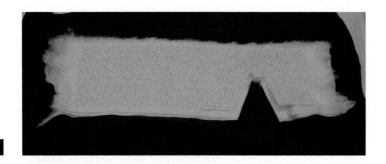

FIGURE
1-29

Radial Gutter Splint

Indication

Similar to the ulnar gutter splint, the radial gutter splint is used for immobilization of the MCP, PIP, and DIP joints, typically for injuries of the metacarpals and proximal phalanges. It is better suited for the index and middle fingers. Additionally, it is effective in immobilizing volar–dorsal and radial–ulnar motion of the wrist and a portion of the forearm. Complete rotational control is not achieved because the proximal radioulnar joint is not immobilized.

Description of Procedure

- Use the patient's unaffected arm to approximate the length of the splint. The appropriate length extends from the fingertips along the radial boarder of the hand, wrist, and forearm to just distal to the elbow.
- At the appropriate position, cut a hole large enough to allow passage of the thumb. The hole may need to be larger than initially appreciated because the splint should sit flat against the hand and wrist to allow motion of the thumb MCP joint (Fig. 1-30).
- Apply sufficient cast padding (see "Cast Padding" section discussed previously).
- With the DIPs, PIPs, and MCPs in extension and the wrist in neutral flexion/extension, apply the splinting material (Fig. 1-31).
- Wrap with bias.
- Maintain extension at the DIPs and PIPs while flexing the MCPs to 90° (Fig. 1-32).

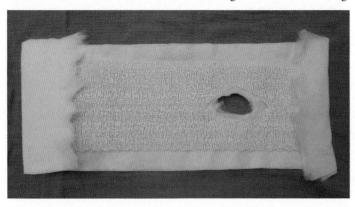

FIGURE
1-30

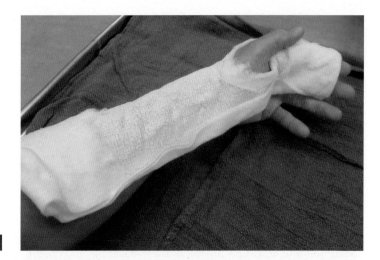

FIGURE
1-31

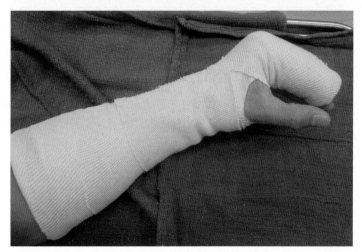

FIGURE
1-32

Short Arm Cast with Outrigger

Indication

Similar to the gutter splints, an outrigger extension on a short arm cast allows immobilization of the DIP, PIP, and MCP joints of the index, middle, ring, and small fingers. It is typically applied for injuries of the metacarpals and proximal phalanges. The short arm cast component also achieves coronal and sagittal plane immobilization of the wrist and a portion of the forearm without achieving complete rotational control because the proximal radioulnar joint is not immobilized.

Description of Procedure

▪ Apply a short arm cast (see "Short Arm Cast" above), leaving the cast two layers thinner than usual.

- Contour an aluminum foam splint to the desired final immobilization position of the finger. Typically, the DIP and PIP joints are maintained in extension, while the MCP joint is placed in 70° to 90° flexion. Usually, the aluminum foam splint will be applied volar aspect but can also be applied dorsally (Fig. 1-33).
- Cut the aluminum foam such that it extends from the tip of the finger to approximately half way down the forearm component of the cast.
- Hold the aluminum foam splint in position and overwrap the final layers of the cast. It is important to keep the bent portion of the aluminum foam splint at or just proximal to the first palmar crease; otherwise, it will not be possible to flex the MCP joint (Fig. 1-34).
- Once the casting material has set, flex the MCP joint to 70° to 90° and secure the finger to the splint with cloth, plastic, or silk tape (Fig. 1-35).

Tips and Other Considerations

- If rotational control of the finger is needed, incorporation of the adjacent, uninjured finger with an additional aluminum foam splint and buddy taping can be helpful.

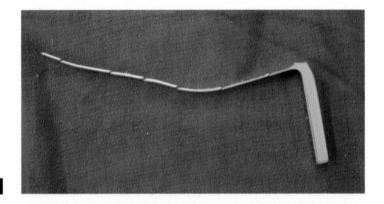

FIGURE
1-33

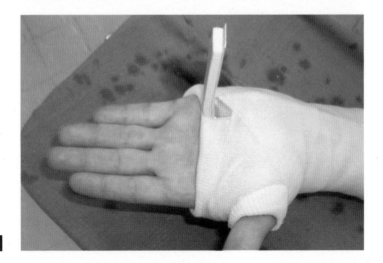

FIGURE
1-34

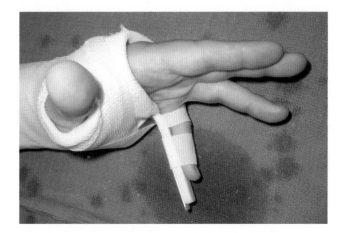

FIGURE
1-35

Thumb Spica Splint

Indication

The thumb spica splint is effective in immobilization of the thumb IP, MCP, and CMC joint as well as some coronal plane, sagittal plane, and rotational control of the wrist and forearm. It is frequently applied in the setting of fractures and dislocations involving the scaphoid, thumb metacarpal, and thumb proximal phalanx.

Description of Procedure

- With a splint, the plaster or fiberglass should not be completely circumferential around the thumb. Three-inch splinting material is commonly used. If necessary, trim the distal portion of the splinting material to obtain this effect. If circumferential immobilization is desired, use a thumb spica cast (see below).
- Use the patient's unaffected arm to approximate the length of the splint. The appropriate length extends from the tip of the thumb along the radial boarder of the hand, wrist, and forearm to just distal to the elbow (Fig. 1-36).

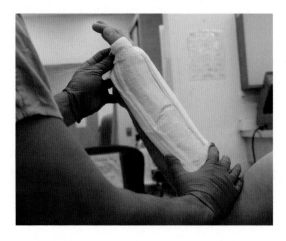

FIGURE
1-36

- Apply sufficient cast padding (see "Cast Padding" section discussed previously).
- Apply the splint material.
- Wrap with bias (Fig. 1-37).

Tips and Other Considerations

- It is typically easier to apply padding as sheets along the inside of the splinting material.
- If using standard three- or four-inch bias, a partial transverse cut with each pass around the thumb will facilitate application.

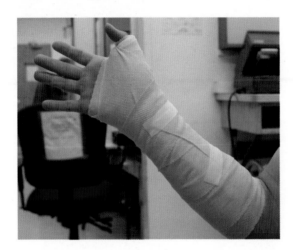

FIGURE
1-37

Thumb Spica Cast

Indication

As with the thumb spica splint, the thumb spica cast is effective in immobilization of the thumb IP, MCP, and CMC joint. It can be incorporated into a short or long arm cast, and, as such, achieves control of the wrist, forearm, elbow, and humerus depending on which level is selected. It is frequently applied in the setting of fractures and dislocations involving the scaphoid, thumb metacarpal, and thumb proximal phalanx.

Description of Procedure

- Apply sufficient cast padding (see "Cast Padding" section discussed previously).
- Using a two-inch roll of casting material, begin at the wrist and extend distally. The thumb IP joint can be incorporated or left free, depending on the level of the injury (Fig. 1-38).
- After sufficient casting material has been applied to the thumb and wrist, begin at the wrist with three-inch rolls and extend to a short or long arm cast, based upon preference and the level of the injury.
- Maintenance of consistent thumb, wrist, forearm, and elbow position during the application of the cast is essential, as manipulation of these joints after the plaster or fiberglass has been applied will create wrinkles or distortion of the casting material that can become pressure points, placing the patient at risk for ulceration.
- While the plaster or fiberglass is still pliable, apply and hold the desired mold (Fig. 1-39).

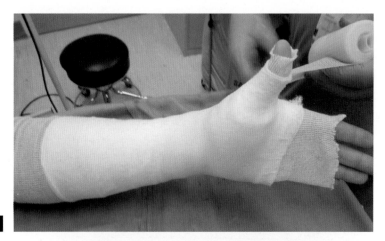

FIGURE
1-38

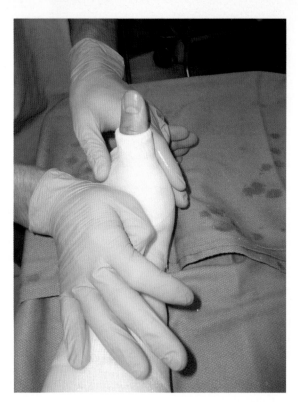

FIGURE
1-39

Tips and Other Considerations

■ A one-inch roll of cast padding is helpful for the thumb. Most facilities do not routinely stock this size; however, it can be made using a scalpel and a large roll (Figs. 1-40 and 1-41).

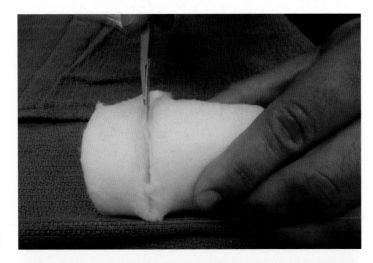

FIGURE
1-40

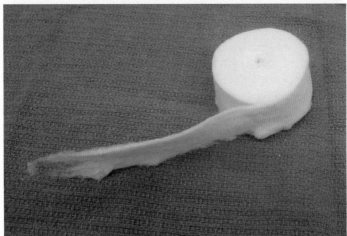

FIGURE
1-41

PIP and DIP Extension Splints

Indication

Extension splints of the finger are used for immobilization of the DIP or PIP joint either in isolation or in conjunction with the other. The DIP extension splint is commonly used for the mallet finger injury (extensor tendon avulsion from the distal phalanx) or volar PIP dislocation (implied central slip avulsion from the middle phalanx).

Description of Procedure

- Use heavy scissors to cut an aluminum foam splint to the desired length. The length of the splint should not interfere with adjacent joints.
- To maintain full extension, the splint often needs to be bent into subtle hyperextension.
- Tape into position on the finger (Fig. 1-42).

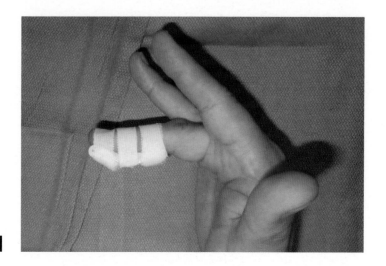

FIGURE
1-42

Tips and Other Considerations

■ To create a more comfortable splint and avoid the risk of skin irritation, cut the metal portion to the desired final length while leaving the foam portion slightly longer at each end. Wrap the foam portion round the sharp, metal cut surface and tape in position.

THE LOWER EXTREMITY

Long Leg Posterior Splint

Indication

A long leg posterior splint is effective in immobilization of foot, ankle, leg, knee, and a portion of the thigh. It is frequently used for fractures or dislocations involving the distal femur, knee, and tibia.

Description of Procedure

■ Use the patient's unaffected leg to approximate the length of the splint. Distally, the splint should begin at the tip of the toes. If the toes are to be left free, begin proximal enough to prevent irritation to the toes during flexion. Extend the splint as far proximal on the thigh as possible (Fig. 1-43).
■ Apply sufficient cast padding (see "Cast Padding" section discussed previously).
■ Apply splinting material.
■ Wrap with bias (Fig. 1-44).

Tips and Other Considerations

■ The appropriate position of the knee and ankle are dictated by the injury. For example, the ankle should be left in gravity plantar flexion for most tibia fractures, as dorsiflexion will cause recurvatum displacement of the fracture; however, with most ankle fracture injuries, effort should be made to immobilize the ankle in dorsiflexion.

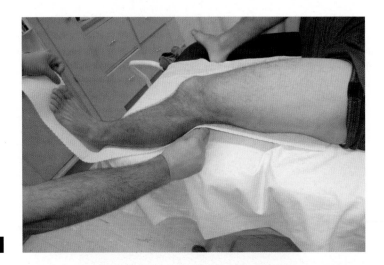

FIGURE
1-43

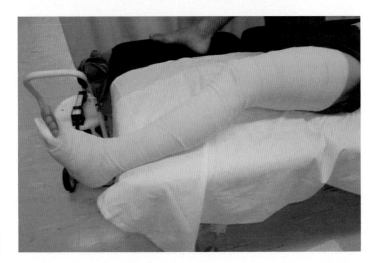

FIGURE
1-44

Long Leg Cast

Indication

As with a long leg posterior splint, a long leg cast is effective in immobilization of foot, ankle, leg, knee, and a portion of the thigh. It is frequently used for fractures or dislocations involving the distal femur, knee, and tibia.

Description of Procedure

- Apply sufficient cast padding (see "Cast Padding" section discussed previously).
- Begin wrapping just proximal to the MTP joints with a four-inch roll. As the cast is extended above the ankle, use a five-inch roll.

■ Maintenance of consistent ankle and knee position during the application of the cast is essential, as manipulation of these joints after the plaster or fiberglass has been applied will create wrinkles or distortion of the casting material that can become pressure points, placing the patient at risk for ulceration.

■ Terminate as far proximal on the thigh as possible (Fig. 1-45).

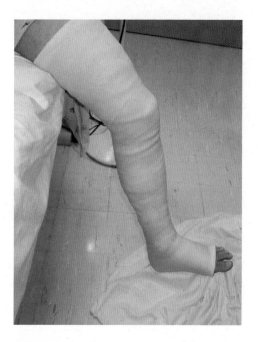

FIGURE
1-45

Tips and Other Considerations

■ An assistant is extremely helpful while applying the cast; however, if an assistant is unavailable, there are two methods for one-provider application.

 ■ The first requires positioning of the patient at the edge of the bed to allow the limb to hang over the bed. If done properly, this position allows access to the foot, ankle, leg, knee, and thigh (Fig. 1-46).

 ■ The second involves a two staged application of the cast. First, apply a short leg cast (see "Short Leg Cast"), leaving some uncovered cast padding at the proximal portion of the cast. After the short leg cast has been appropriately molded and has hardened, change position to allow access to the thigh. Extend the cast padding above the knee; do not wrap cast padding over the plaster or fiberglass on the leg that has already hardened (this will prevent the extended casting material from adhering to the short leg cast). Next, extend the casting material above the knee. In order to avoid a weak transition point, begin wrapping cast material far distal to the transition point.

■ The appropriate position of the knee and ankle are dictated by the injury. For example, the ankle should be left in gravity plantar flexion for most tibia fractures, as dorsiflexion will cause recurvatum displacement of the fracture; however, with most ankle fracture injuries, effort should be made to immobilize the ankle in dorsiflexion.

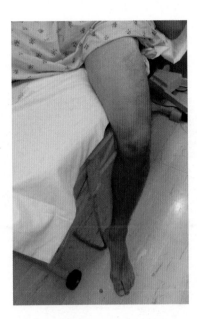

FIGURE
1-46

Cylinder Cast

Indication

A cylinder cast is useful for immobilization of the knee and a portion of both the thigh and the leg. It is most commonly used for injuries of the extensor mechanism of the knee.

Description of Procedure

- Apply sufficient cast padding (see "Cast Padding" section discussed previously).
- Apply casting material. It is acceptable to begin proximally or distally.
- Distally, the cast should terminate about the medial and lateral malleolus. Proximally the cast should extend as far as possible (Fig. 1-47).

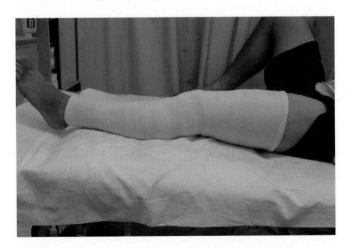

FIGURE
1-47

- The knee should be maintained in full but not hyperextension while the cast is setting.
- Good medial and lateral femoral condyle, patellar, and supramalleolar molds are crucial to avoid slipping and irritation of the cast (Fig. 1-48).

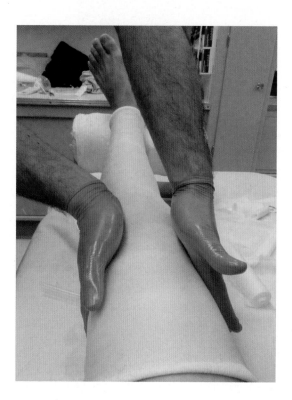

FIGURE
1-48

Short Leg Posterior Splint

Indication

A short leg posterior splint is effective in immobilization of the foot, ankle, and a portion of the leg. It is frequently used for fractures of the distal tibial plafond, ankle, and foot.

Description of Procedure

- Use the patient's unaffected leg to approximate the length of the splint. Distally, the splint should begin at the tip of the toes. If the toes are to be left free, begin proximal enough to prevent irritation to the toes during flexion. Proximally, extend the splint as far proximal on the calf as possible yet distal enough to avoid impingement of the cast on the popliteal fossa during knee flexion (Fig. 1-49).
- Apply sufficient cast padding (see "Cast Padding" section discussed previously).
- Apply splint material.
- Wrap with bias (Fig. 1-50).
- Ensure that popliteal impingement will not occur with knee flexion (Fig. 1-51).

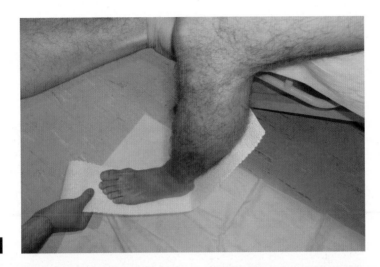

FIGURE
1-49

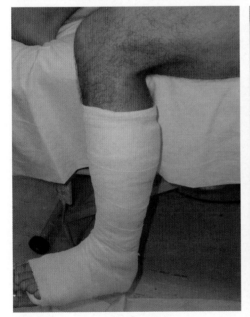

FIGURE
1-50

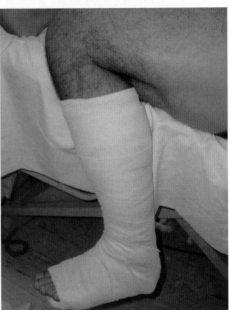

FIGURE
1-51

Tips and Other Considerations

■ The appropriate position of the ankle is dictated by the injury. For example, the ankle should be left in gravity plantar flexion for most tibia fractures, as dorsiflexion will cause recurvatum displacement of the fracture; however, with most ankle fracture injuries, effort should be made to immobilize the ankle in dorsiflexion.

Short Leg Cast

Indication

A short leg cast is effective in immobilization of the foot, ankle, and a portion of the leg. It is frequently used for fractures of the distal tibial plafond, ankle, and foot.

Description of Procedure

- Apply sufficient cast padding (see "Cast Padding" section discussed previously).
- Begin wrapping just proximal to the MTP joints with a four-inch roll. As the cast is extended above the ankle, use a five-inch roll (Fig. 1-52).
- Maintenance of consistent ankle position during the application of the cast is essential, as manipulation after the plaster or fiberglass has been applied will create wrinkles or distortion of the casting material that can become pressure points, placing the patient at risk for ulceration.

Tips and Other Considerations

- The appropriate position of the ankle is dictated by the injury. For example, the ankle should be left in gravity plantar flexion for most tibia fractures, as dorsiflexion will cause recurvatum displacement of the fracture; however, with most ankle fracture injuries, effort should be made to immobilize the ankle in dorsiflexion.

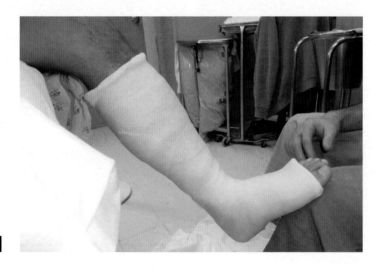

FIGURE
1-52

Bulky Jones Splint

Indication

The Bulky Jones splint is effective for immobilization of the foot, ankle, and a portion of the leg. The theory behind a Bulky Jones splint is that an excessive amount of soft cast padding under a compressive dressing will provide a longer lasting gentle soft tissue compression because as swelling decreases with time, the padding will expand and continue to provide a gentle compressive environment. For this reason, it is commonly used for high-energy injuries such as fractures of the tibial plafond or calcaneus.

Description of Procedure

- Use the patient's unaffected leg to approximate the length of the splint. For the posterior slab, the length is identical to a short leg posterior splint (see above). For the "U" portion of the splint, the proximal extent should be at the fibular head and its medial equivalent while wrapping around the midfoot, not the hindfoot, with the front portion of the "U" along the metatarsal heads (Figs. 1-53 and 1-54).
- Use the softest cast padding available at your facility. Apply in a very thick layer, followed by a later of bias under moderate, but not excessive, compression (Figs. 1-55 and 1-56).
- Apply splinting material as described above. It is typically easiest to apply the posterior slab first, followed by the "U" portion.
- Wrap with bias (Fig. 1-57).

Tips and Other Considerations

- The appropriate position of the knee and ankle are dictated by the injury. For example, the ankle should be left in gravity plantar flexion for most tibia fractures, as dorsiflexion will cause recurvatum displacement of the fracture; however, with most ankle fracture injuries, effort should be made to immobilize the ankle in dorsiflexion.

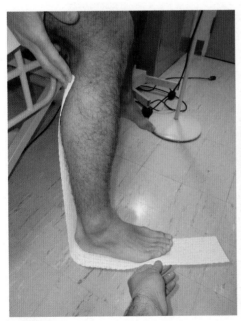

FIGURE
1-53

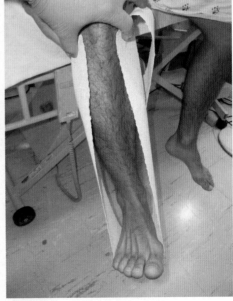

FIGURE
1-54

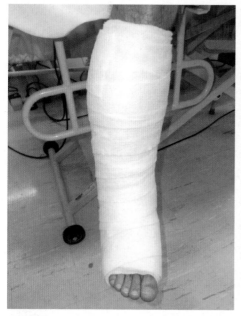

FIGURE
1-55

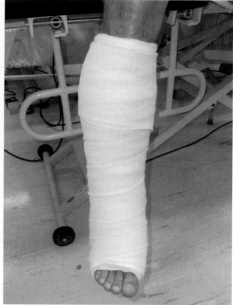

FIGURE
1-56

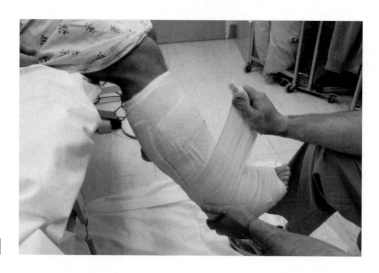

FIGURE
1-57

FIGURE CREDITS

Figure 1-14   From Wenger DR, Pring ME, Rang M. *Rang's Children's Fractures*. 3rd ed. Philadelphia, PA: Lippincott Williams & Wilkins; 2005.

The Shoulder and Arm

INJECTIONS AND ASPIRATIONS

Glenohumeral Injection: Anterior Approach

Indication

The intraarticular placement of a needle in the glenohumeral joint allows for diagnostic aspiration, anesthesia for reduction maneuvers, and administration of medications (e.g., corticosteroids).

Description of Procedure

- Position the patient supine or comfortably sitting (our preference).
- Prepare the skin with an antimicrobial agent such as alcohol, Betadine, or chlorhexidine gluconate (our preference).
- The minimum length of needle is 1.5 inches. Since a large amount of soft tissue surrounds the shoulder, when in doubt use a spinal needle. The gauge of needle depends on the procedure: larger bore (18G to 20G) for aspirations and smaller for injections (22G to 25G).
- *Optional:* The overlying skin is anesthetized with 2 to 3 cc of 1% lidocaine using a 25G to 30G needle. The use of local anesthetic is debatable. Some physicians feel it is not helpful because only the skin will be anesthetized, and a second injection is required. We do not routinely use local anesthetic prior to skin penetration. However, the needle should penetrate the skin quickly to minimize pain.
- The entry site is found 1 cm lateral to the coracoid process and medial to the lesser tuberosity. Typically, the clinician feels a "pop" as the needle traverses the anterior capsule (Fig. 2-1).
- Completely bury a 1.5-inch needle and aspirate to obtain synovial fluid confirming that you are in the joint. Depending on the procedure, continue to aspirate the necessary amount of fluid or inject medication.

Tips and Other Considerations

- Traditionally, 1 cm lateral to the coracoid has been used as the entry site, but we have had improved accuracy entering immediately lateral to the coracoid (Fig. 2-2).

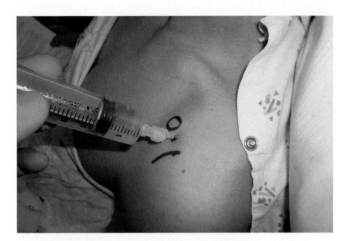

FIGURE
2-1

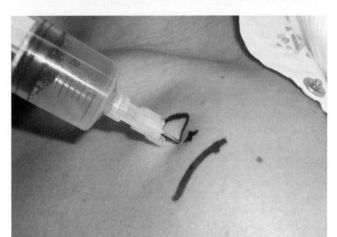

FIGURE
2-2

Glenohumeral Injection: Posterior Approach

Indication

Clinical preference guides approach. In the case of overlying cellulitis, always choose the approach furthest from the affected area to avoid iatrogenic contamination of the joint.

Description of Procedure

- Position the patient in a seated posture to allow access to the posterior portion of the shoulder. If the patient is unable to sit, then position lateral decubitus with the affected shoulder up.
- Again a 1.5-inch needle is the minimum length needed, and a longer needle is used for larger patients. For this injection, we always use a spinal needle due to the large amount of soft tissue covering the posterior aspect of the glenohumeral joint.

- The entry site is the posterior shoulder 2 cm inferior and 1 cm medial to the posterolateral tip of the acromion. Always direct the needle toward the tip of the coracoid process for accurate placement into the glenohumeral joint (Fig. 2-3).
- Aspirate a small amount of synovial fluid to confirm placement and continue with aspiration or injection.

Tips and Other Considerations

- A "soft spot" exists overlying the posterior glenohumeral joint and is an excellent way to confirm that you have a good starting point (Fig. 2-4).

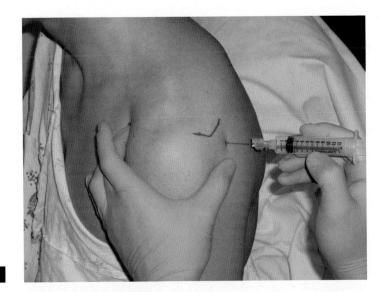

FIGURE
2-3

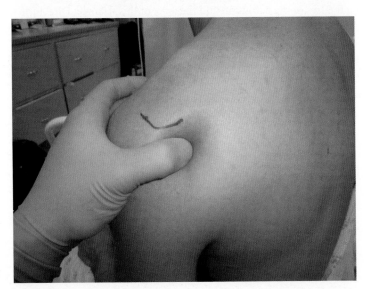

FIGURE
2-4

- Use your free hand to palpate the tip of the coracoid process anteriorly to assist in guiding the needle into the joint space. By aiming the needle toward your digit on the coracoid, you will increase the accuracy of placement.

Subacromial Injection

Indication

A subacromial injection is commonly used to treat degenerative conditions of the shoulder, including impingement syndrome/bursitis and rotator cuff pathology.

Description of Procedure

- Position the patient in a seated posture to allow access to the posterior portion of the shoulder. If the patient is unable to sit, then position lateral decubitus with the affected shoulder up.
- Typically a 1.5-inch needle is the sufficient to access the subacromial space.
- The entry site is the posterior shoulder 2 cm inferior and 1 cm medial to the posterolateral tip of the acromion.
- The needle is directed cephalad into the subacromial space. We place our free hand on the acromioclavicular joint and aim just lateral to this point. Once the needle has pierced the skin, direct it just under the acromion toward the acromioclavicular joint (Fig. 2-5).
- The injection should flow easily. If resistance is felt, redirect the needle as it may be embedded in the rotator cuff.

Tips and Other Considerations

- A soft spot exists just inferior and medial to the posterolateral tip of the acromion, which marks the entry point for the subacromial space.
- An additional access point to the subacromial space is lateral. To find this, mark the anterior and posterior tips of the acromion. Next palpate the triangular depression between the clavicle, acromion, and scapular spine. The entry point exists at a spot bisected by a line connecting the tips of the acromion and the apex of this triangle. Direct the needle under the acromion and inject in a similar fashion to the posterior approach (Fig. 2-6).

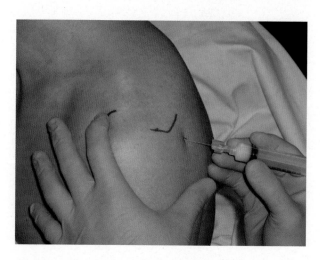

FIGURE

2-5

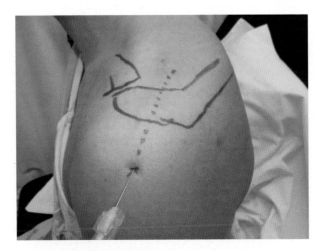

FIGURE
2-6

Acromioclavicular Joint Injection

Indication

The insertion of a needle in the acromioclavicular (AC) joint is used for the treatment of AC joint arthritis, differentiating pain originating from the AC joint from other shoulder pathology, and more rarely to obtain synovial fluid for analysis.

Description of Procedure

- Position the patient in a seated posture. Since the AC joint is small, a 22G needle is used to aid in tactile feedback. With experience, a finer needle can be used to enter the joint.
- To locate the entry site, palpate the distal clavicle until a small depression is felt; this is the AC joint. The entry site is the superior aspect of the AC joint just above this depression. With a slight lateral-to-medial inclination, the needle pierces the skin and joint capsule (Fig. 2-7).

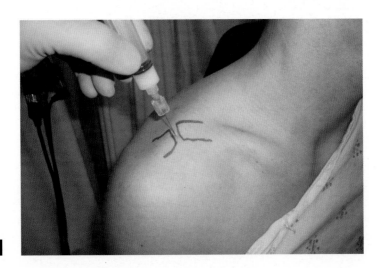

FIGURE
2-7

Tips and Other Considerations

- Positioning the patient's arm behind the back opens the anterior portion of the AC joint, which can make it easier to palpate and enter (Fig. 2-8).
- If the needle is advanced too far, it is possible to pierce the inferior AC joint capsule entering the subacromial space.

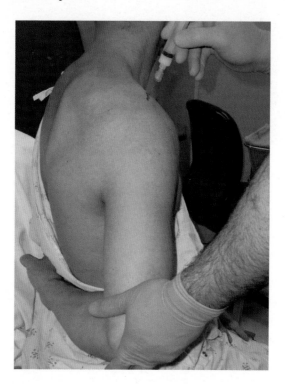

FIGURE
2-8

CLOSED REDUCTIONS

Anterior Glenohumeral Joint Dislocation

Indication

Acute anterior glenohumeral dislocations can be treated successfully with a variety of closed reduction maneuvers. Glenohumeral dislocations greater than 4 weeks old should be treated with caution, because they are at a higher risk of postreduction instability, fracture, and injury to neurovascular structures. For these reasons, we limit closed reduction in the emergency room to dislocations less than 4 weeks old.

Description of Procedure

Regardless of the specific technique used, patient relaxation and comfort are paramount. Our preference is to perform the reduction maneuver after administering a single dose of narcotic and an intraarticular injection of lidocaine into the glenohumeral joint. Alternatively, conscious sedation with any variety of medications can be used.

TRACTION–COUNTERTRACTION

■ Position the patient supine. Place a sheet under the patient's affected axilla and wrap it around the thorax.

■ An assistant standing on the opposite side of the table holds both ends of the sheet to provide countertraction (Fig. 2-9).

■ Grasp the patient's arm and provide gentle inline traction and external rotation. A palpable clunk may be felt as the humeral head reduces (Fig. 2-10).

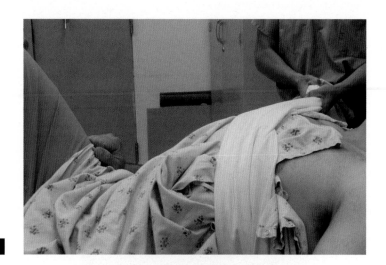

FIGURE
2-9

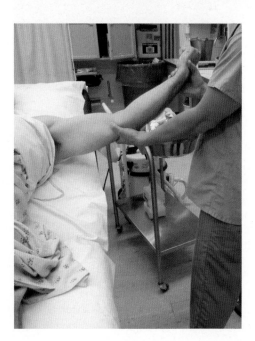

FIGURE
2-10

Stimson Technique[1]

- Position the patient prone. Place a strap around the patient to ensure the patient does not fall off the gurney if you plan to leave the bedside during the reduction.
- With the affected arm hanging over the side of the bed, attach 10 lb of weight to the patient's wrist (Fig. 2-11).
- In 10 to 15 minutes, return to the bedside to confirm reduction of the glenohumeral joint. If the reduction has not occurred, then externally rotate the arm and perform scapular manipulation (described in next section).

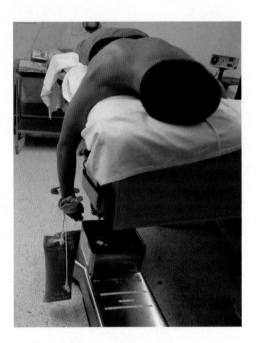

FIGURE
2-11

Scapular Manipulation Technique

- For this technique, the patient can be positioned prone, supine, or lateral decubitus. We prefer to combine this technique with the Stimpson technique. Therefore, the patient is positioned prone, and weight is used to relax the muscles surrounding the shoulder girdle.
- The arm is placed in 90° of forward flexion and slowly manipulated into maximal external rotation. Next the superior aspect of the scapula is grasped and stabilized with one hand. The thumb of the contralateral hand is then placed at the inferior pole of the scapula, and a medially directed force is applied. This positions the scapula in an ideal position for reduction to occur (Fig. 2-12).

External Rotation Technique (Modified Kocher)

- Position the patient in a seated posture. One hand is used to stabilize the arm against the chest wall and in slight forward flexion. Forward flexion allows for relaxation of anterior structures such as the capsule, conjoint tendon, and long head of the biceps.

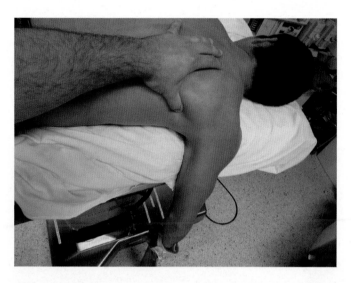

FIGURE

2-12

- The contralateral hand grasps the patient's wrist and slowly externally rotates the arm. If the patient experiences discomfort, the rate of external rotation is slowed. Although not initially described, to achieve reduction, gentle longitudinal traction may be necessary. Often the humeral head reduces during the external rotation maneuver (Fig. 2-13).
- Internal rotation places the humeral head in contact with the glenoid, completing the reduction.

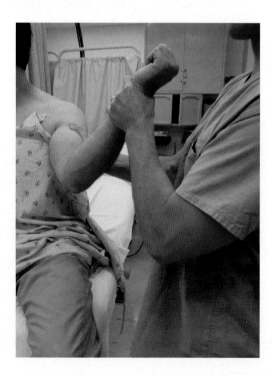

FIGURE

2-13

Milch Technique[2]

- The patient is positioned supine. The arm is slowly abducted to lie fully overhead. This allows all muscles to become coaxial with the humerus. With the free hand, grasp the clavicle and superior scapula with your digits and place your thumb under the dislocated humeral head (Fig. 2-14).
- Once fully overhead, simultaneously pull gentle traction, while using your thumb to reduce the humeral head over the glenoid rim.

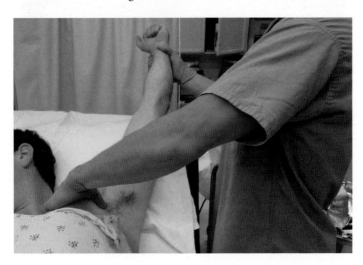

FIGURE
2-14

Spaso Technique[3]

- The patient is positioned supine. The arm is forward flexed to 90° so that the arm is in a vertical position. Once the arm is vertical, pull traction straight up toward the ceiling (Fig. 2-15).

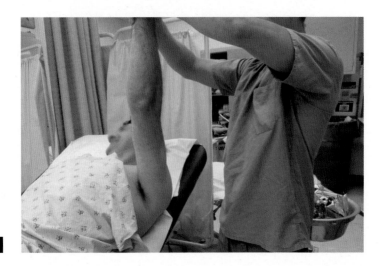

FIGURE
2-15

- Gentle external rotation completes the reduction.
- If the shoulder does not undergo reduction initially, then an assistant can manipulate the humeral head into the glenoid.
- A sign of insufficient analgesia is if the patient voluntarily lifts the scapula off the examination table (Fig. 2-16).

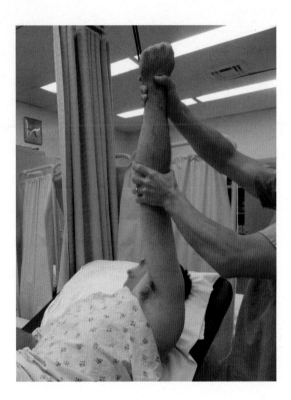

FIGURE
2-16

AUTHOR'S PREFERRED TECHNIQUE

- Position the patient supine, with a sheet wrapped around the patient's thorax.
- Forward flex and abduct the shoulder 45° in 20° to 30° of external rotation. This relaxes the anterior structures and brings the tuberosities away from the glenoid rim.
- Gently pull inline traction with your outside hand grasping the distal humeral condyles. An assistant is helpful to apply countertraction via the thorax sheet.
- Use your inside hand to grasp the medial arm within the axilla. This hand gently manipulates the humeral head from underneath the glenoid rim. It also guides the head back into the glenoid (Fig. 2-17).

Tips and Other Considerations

- We recommend performing a shoulder trauma series both prior to and after any reduction technique to document preexisting fractures and accuracy of reduction. This includes a true AP, scapular-Y, and axillary view of the shoulder.

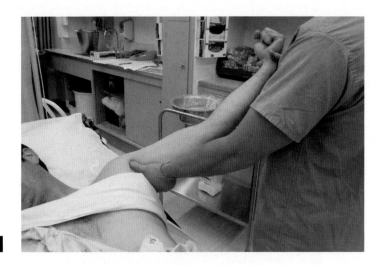

FIGURE
2-17

- Nearly all reduction techniques for anterior shoulder dislocations require two maneuvers: (1) external rotation to appose the articular surfaces and maneuver the tuberosities away from the glenoid rim and (2) longitudinal traction.
- Patient comfort is paramount. If the patient is in discomfort, then an alternative method of analgesia must be considered.
- An accurate way to clinically confirm reduction is to palpate under the lateral acromion. If the humeral head is dislocated, then an empty space will be felt. If the glenohumeral joint is reduced, the humeral head is easily felt occupying this space.
- The optimal position of immobilization is controversial. If the reduction is stable, then we typically place the patient in a simple sling. Some clinicians immobilize the patient in external rotation using a splint or prefabricated shoulder immobilizer, which some think decreases the risk of redislocation.

Posterior Glenohumeral Joint Dislocation

Indication

Posterior glenohumeral dislocations comprise a minority of acute shoulder dislocations; however, they are more commonly missed than their anterior counterpart. A high index of suspicion is necessary in the diagnosis, particularly in the setting of high-energy trauma and seizures. Clinically, the arm is held in internal rotation, with a block to external rotation.

Description of Procedure

- The patient is placed supine. It is critical to maximally adduct and internally rotate the shoulder while pulling gentle traction to unlock the humeral head from the glenoid rim.
- Once the shoulder is unlocked, the arm is gradually externally rotated until a reduction is palpated. At this point, abduction can also help reduce the joint.
- A shoulder immobilizer is applied. When the joint is unstable after reduction, we will immobilize the shoulder in external rotation (see anterior glenohumeral joint).

Tips and Other Considerations

- Do not proceed with external rotation of the shoulder until the humeral head is disengaged (unlocked) from the glenoid rim. Premature external rotation can lead to fracture.
- If there is difficulty with unlocking the humeral head, then either have an assistant grasp the medial aspect of the proximal arm within the axilla and provide lateral traction or wrap a sheet around the upper arm for lateral traction.

Inferior Glenohumeral Joint Dislocation/Luxatio Erecta

Indication

Inferior glenohumeral dislocations are rare, but the clinical presentation is striking because the patient presents with the arm fixed in an overhead position. To reduce inferior glenohumeral dislocations, the first goal is to convert it to an anterior dislocation followed by standard anterior dislocation reduction techniques.

Description of Procedure

- The patient is placed supine. Conscious sedation is frequently required.
- The first step is to convert the inferior dislocation into an anterior dislocation. To accomplish this, gently pull superior traction while using the other hand to manipulate the humeral head along the anterior glenoid rim. The humeral head is often palpable on the chest wall and easily directed laterally and anteriorly.
- Once the humeral head is properly positioned anterior to the glenoid, bring the arm from its abducted position to an adducted position. In other words, bring it from overhead to by the patient's side.
- Now proceed with reduction of the anterior shoulder dislocation as described above.
- Place a sling.

Tips and Other Considerations

- It is important to perform a careful postreduction neurovascular exam. Inferior shoulder dislocations have the highest rates of neurovascular injury, particularly to the axillary nerve.

Proximal Humerus Fracture

Indication

In adults, we rarely manipulate a proximal humerus fracture. It is both difficult to obtain and maintain a reduction with nonsurgical treatment. Typically, we will place the patient in a sling if the injury films are acceptable or embark on surgical treatment if they are not. However, occasionally we are presented with a displaced surgical neck fracture with an intact medial calcar, which can be improved with a reduction maneuver. We do not attempt to reduce the tuberosities.

Description of Procedure

- The major deforming forces are the supraspinatus pulling the head fragment into varus (if tuberosities intact) and the pectoralis major displacing the humeral shaft medially and anteriorly with an internal rotation moment. The reduction maneuver is primarily based on relaxing the pectoralis major.

■ The patient is positioned supine, with the head of the bed elevated 30°. The arm is initially flexed, adducted and internally rotated, which relaxes the pectoralis major.

■ One hand is used to pull longitudinal traction while the other hand manipulates the humeral shaft. Typically, the shaft is moved lateral and posterior to contact the humeral head. The arm is then slowly externally rotated to correct the external rotation deformity (Fig. 2-18).

■ A shoulder immobilizer is applied.

Tips and Other Considerations

■ Prior to reduction of a proximal humerus fracture, obtain upright radiographs. Often, the simple application of gravity will result in acceptable alignment of two-part proximal humerus fractures. The patient can then be treated nonoperatively in an upright position (e.g., sleep in a recliner chair) until early fracture healing is present (typically 2 to 4 weeks).

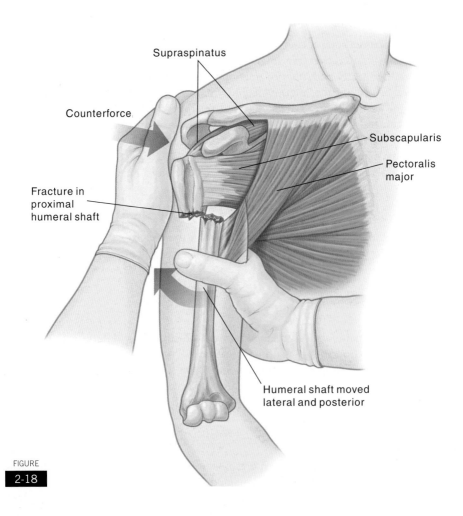

FIGURE

2-18

■ Approach combined fracture dislocations of the proximal humerus with caution. Reduction attempts are usually unsuccessful and may further compromise the blood supply to the humeral head.

Sternoclavicular Joint Dislocation

Indication

Anterior sternoclavicular dislocations can be reduced in the emergency room but are rarely stable. Chronic anterior dislocation rarely results in functional impairment. Anterior and posterior subluxations usually do not require a reduction, and the joint is simply protected with a figure-of-eight brace.

Posterior sternoclavicular joint dislocations are more concerning and should be reduced. Prior to reduction, the patient should be asked about symptoms of dyspnea or dysphagia, and a careful neurovascular exam documented. An emergent reduction may be necessary in cases involving compression of the trachea, esophagus, brachial plexus, or great vessels.

Description of Procedure

■ Prior to the reduction of a posterior sternoclavicular dislocation, a thoracic surgeon should be contacted and be on standby in case of great vessel injury. Some centers will prep and drape the chest and have cardiothoracic instruments in the operating room prior to performing a closed reduction since great vessel rupture may result in rapid exsanguination.

■ We always perform this reduction under general anesthesia to allow immediate thoracotomy in the case of great vessel injury.

■ The patient is positioned supine. A minimum of 4-inch thick sandbag or towel roll is placed between the shoulders. The arm is abducted to 90° and inline traction is initiated. Often a significant amount of traction is necessary to dislodge the clavicle from the posterior manubrium (Figs. 2-19 and 2-20).

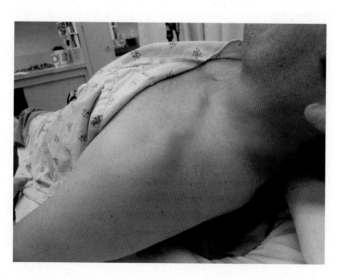

FIGURE
2-19

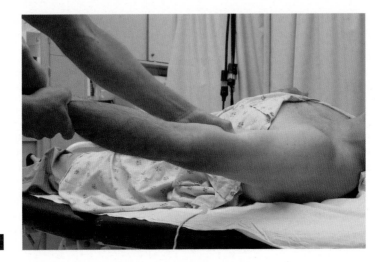

FIGURE
2-20

- If reduction does not occur, then a second surgeon grasps the clavicle and manipulates it anteriorly.
- If this is not successful, we place a small pointed reduction tenaculum around the proximal clavicle and pull it anteriorly (Fig. 2-21).
- A figure-of-eight brace is placed.

Tips and Other Considerations

- A towel clamp is often too flimsy; therefore, we use the sturdier small-pointed reduction tenaculum. We have had instances of a towel clamp bending or losing purchase.
- The medial physis of the clavicle is the last to fuse; therefore, a physeal injury must be suspected in patients younger than 25 years old. However, the reduction maneuver is unchanged.

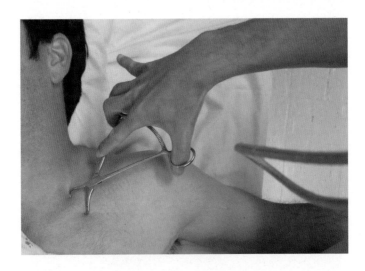

FIGURE
2-21

Clavicular Fracture

Indication

The indications for surgical treatment of clavicular fractures are evolving. Currently, we rarely manipulate clavicular fractures as any reduction is difficult, if not impossible, to maintain until fracture union. Our current practice is to limit closed reduction of clavicular fractures to pediatric patients since the thick periosteum often allows a more stable reduction.

Description of Procedure

■ Have the patient seated with the back accessible. Standing behind the patient, grasp both shoulders. Place a towel over your knee (for padding), and place your knee between the patient's scapulae. Pull back on the shoulders to allow scapular retraction, and push gently forward with your knee (Fig. 2-22).

■ Have an assistant apply a figure-of-eight brace snuggly.

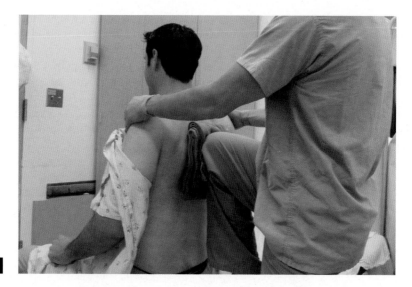

FIGURE
2-22

Tips and Other Considerations

■ The patient must tighten the figure-of-eight brace twice daily to maintain the reduction. Also, you must warn the patient to observe for brace complications including skin breakdown and symptoms of brachial plexus or axillary vessel compression.

■ A figure-of-eight brace is designed to maintain a reduction, but is often uncomfortable. If no reduction is attempted, then a sling is more comfortable for the patient.

■ A reduction can also be obtained in the supine position with a method similar to that for posterior sternoclavicular dislocations. However, we perform clavicular reductions seated because it is easier to place the figure-of-eight bandage without losing the reduction.

Humeral Shaft Fracture

Indication

The vast majority of humeral shaft fractures are treated nonsurgically. For displaced fractures, the treatment begins with a closed reduction and immobilization in a coaptation splint. This is followed by fracture brace placement.

Tolerances

Expert opinion parameters of a successful closed reduction of a humeral shaft fracture are ≤20° sagittal plane angulation, ≤30° varus angulation, ≤15° malrotation, and ≤3 cm of shortening.

Description of Procedure

- Typically, closed reduction of a humeral shaft fracture can be performed without sedation after a dose of intravenous pain medicine.
- Position the patient in a seated posture, with the affected arm at the side. The fracture is invariably in varus angulation, but is equally likely to demonstrate apex anterior or posterior angulation. The next step depends on the amount of translation and shortening.
- If minimal translation and shortening are present, then we apply a coaptation splint first and mold the splint to straighten the arm. One hand is placed laterally at the fracture site and the other hand cupping the posteromedial elbow (Fig. 2-23). It is often helpful to have an assistant stabilize the patient's thorax.
- With your hands in this configuration, provide a valgus mold while positioning the elbow anterior or posterior depending on the sagittal plane angulation. Hold the molds until the splint is completely hard.

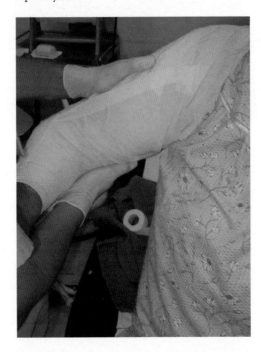

FIGURE
2-23

- If there is translation and shortening, then this must be corrected prior to placement of the splint. Abduct the arm 20° to 30° and use one hand to gently pull traction while an assistant steadies the patient. The other hand gently manipulates the fracture site to align the proximal and distal fragments. After the translation has been reduced, inline traction is maintained. The assistant then places the coaptation splint, and the angulation is corrected in the same fashion as described above.

Tips and Other Considerations

- After a well-molded coaptation splint is placed, to prevent varus settling, we often place a stack of towels at the waist as a bolster for the arm. Alternatively, a commercially available abduction sling more conveniently provides the same effect (Figs. 2-24 and 2-25).
- We judge the time to conversion to a fracture brace based on the patient's comfort level. Once the acute pain and swelling subsides, the fracture brace is placed, typically at 7 to 14 days. It is important for the swelling to subside prior to placement of the fracture brace, because it works by maintaining hydrostatic pressure in the muscles surrounding the fracture.
- The patient should be instructed to sleep in a semireclined position for the first 4 weeks to prevent fracture displacement.
- Another option for initial immobilization is a hanging arm cast. This form of immobilization results in distraction; therefore, we only use it in the rare case of an oblique or spiral fracture with an unacceptable amount of shortening. It is contraindicated in transverse fracture patterns as it results in a high rate of nonunion secondary to excessive distraction.

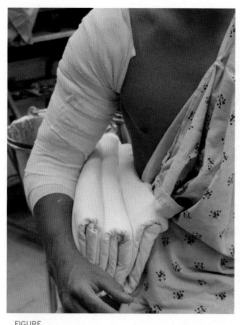
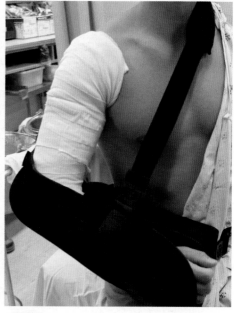

FIGURE
2-24

FIGURE
2-25

■ These methods are best suited for midshaft humerus fractures. Both proximal and distal humeral shaft fractures are amenable but more difficult to treat nonsurgically. In proximal humeral diaphyseal fractures, the medial limb of the coaptation splint often ends at the fracture site resulting in poor initial immobilization. An over-the-shoulder fracture brace (e.g., clamshell extension) can then be used for the second stage of treatment. In distal humeral shaft fractures, braces that extend to the forearm with a hinge for elbow motion can be used.

PEDIATRIC CONSIDERATIONS

Pediatric Proximal Humerus Fracture

Indication

The child's proximal humerus has an impressive ability to remodel. Therefore, most pediatric proximal humerus fractures are treated nonoperatively. The child younger than 10 years with a proximal humerus fracture is nearly always treated nonoperatively. In children older than 13 years, less deformity is accepted (controversial, but most recommend less than 30° to 40° of angulation and 50% displacement). The child from 10 to 13 years old must be treated on an individual-case basis, but typically nonoperative management is appropriate.

Tolerances

■ ≤10 years old: angulation of up to 60° remodels completely.
■ >10 years old: less than 30° angulation in the sagittal and coronal plane.

Description of Procedure

■ The reduction technique for pediatric proximal humerus fractures is similar to that for adults. The primary deforming forces are the pectoralis major and rotator cuff musculature.
■ The reduction maneuver is started in internal rotation and adduction with traction to realign the arm.
■ Next the arm is brought into abduction and external rotation to complete the reduction.
■ If apex anterior angulation persists, then a palm on the anterior proximal arm usually results in correction of the sagittal plane deformity.

Tips and Other Considerations

■ Soft tissue impediments to closed reduction include the biceps tendon and periosteal flaps.

REFERENCES

1. Stimson LA. An easy method of reducing dislocations of the shoulder and hip. *Med Rec.* 1900;57:356–357.
2. Milch H. The treatment of recent dislocations and fracture dislocations of the shoulder. *J. Bone Joint Surg.* 1949;31:173–180.
3. Yuen MC, Yap PG, Chan YT, et al. An easy method to reduce anterior shoulder dislocation: the Spaso technique. *Emerg Med J.* 2001;18:370–372.

The Elbow and Forearm

INJECTIONS AND ASPIRATIONS

Elbow Joint Injection

Indication

The intraarticular placement of a needle in the elbow joint allows for diagnostic aspiration, anesthesia for reduction maneuvers and evaluation of mechanical blocks to motion, and administration of therapeutics (e.g., corticosteroids).

Description of Procedure

■ Position the patient either supine or seated depending on which position is more comfortable for the patient. The elbow can be in any position, but a position of slight (~45°) flexion is optimal.

■ Prepare the skin with an antimicrobial agent such as alcohol, Betadine, or chlorhexidine gluconate (our preference).

■ *Optional:* The overlying skin is anesthetized with 2 to 3 cc of 1% lidocaine without epinephrine using a 25G to 30G needle. The use of local anesthetic is debatable. Some physicians feel it is not helpful because only the skin will be anesthetized, and a second injection is required. We do not routinely use local anesthetic prior to skin penetration. However, the needle should penetrate the skin quickly to minimize pain.

■ Palpate three structures which form a triangle on the posterolateral aspect of the elbow: the lateral epicondyle, radial head, and lateral tip of olecranon. The soft spot in the center of this triangle is the entry point for the needle (Fig. 3-1).

■ The needle should enter the joint easily, and a small amount of synovial fluid is aspirated to confirm intraarticular placement. If performing an injection, the fluid should enter the joint with little to no resistance.

Tips and Other Considerations

■ Lacerations around the elbow are common. Often, a saline load test is used in the setting of an open wound to evaluate for the presence of a traumatic arthrotomy. To evaluate for a traumatic arthrotomy, inject 50 cc of normal saline (*optional:* use diluted methylene blue for improved visualization) into the joint using the described technique and observe for extravasation of the solution out of the open wound.

■ In the presence of a radial head fracture, it is often difficult to evaluate the elbow for a mechanical block because of guarding secondary to pain. Aspiration of the hematoma and infusion of 5 cc of 1% lidocaine into the elbow joint anesthetizes the elbow, enabling a range of motion examination. This allows the practitioner to distinguish guarding secondary to pain from a mechanical block from intraarticular incongruency.

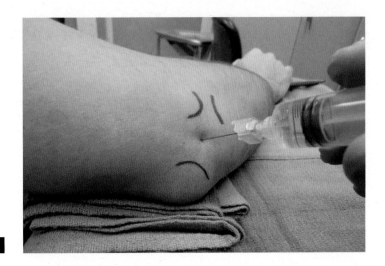

FIGURE

3-1

Olecranon Bursa Aspiration/Injection

Indication

Aspiration is indicated in the diagnosis and treatment of patients with aseptic and septic olecranon bursitis. In aseptic bursitis, the fluid collection is drained, and the clinician has the option of infusing a therapeutic agent (corticosteroid or sclerosing agent). In septic bursitis, needle drainage is used to identify the offending bacteria, and the resulting decompression can provide definitive treatment.

Description of Procedure

- Position the patient supine, with the arm at the patient's side resting on a stack of towels. Prepare the skin with a sterile prep.
- Palpate the fluctuant mass directly over the tip of the olecranon. The needle is inserted into the bursa and the contents are aspirated. Often, the bursa contains septations which must be broken by sweeping the needle through the bursa while intermittently aspirating (Fig. 3-2).
- If infusion of a therapeutic agent is desired, a hemostat is used to stabilize the needle while removing the syringe used to aspirate and replacing it with a syringe loaded with corticosteroid or sclerosing agent.
- A compression bandage should be wrapped snuggly to discourage reaccumulation of fluid.

Tips and Other Considerations

- Do not inject any therapeutic agents (corticosteroid or sclerosing agent) if septic olecranon bursitis is suspected.

Lateral Epicondylitis Injection

Indication

Injections of various therapeutic agents are used to treat lateral epicondylitis if the patient fails conservative treatment.

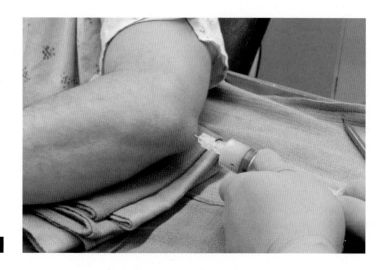

FIGURE
3-2

Description of Procedure

■ The patient is positioned supine with the elbow slightly flexed and pronated. The area of maximal tenderness is identified by the patient, confirmed by palpation, and marked. The skin is prepared in a sterile fashion (Fig. 3-3).
■ At the marked spot, a 22G needle is inserted down to bone and withdrawn 1 mm. The solution is slowly injected (Fig. 3-4).

Tips and Other Considerations

■ A variety of therapeutic agents can be injected. We typically inject 2 ml of 1% lidocaine mixed with 1 ml of methylprednisolone (40 mg/ml). More recently, botulinum toxin, whole blood, and platelet-rich plasma injections have been used to treat lateral epicondylitis.

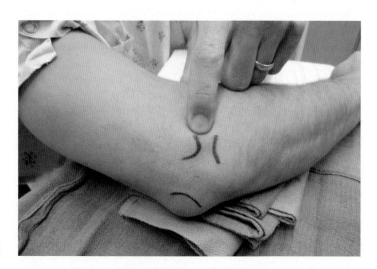

FIGURE
3-3

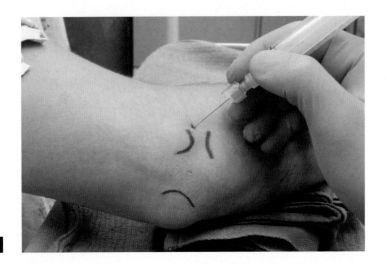

FIGURE

3-4

CLOSED REDUCTIONS

In adults, the majority of displaced fractures and fracture dislocations around the elbow and forearm are treated surgically to provide the best functional outcome. This includes most displaced intraarticular distal humerus, radial head, olecranon, and diaphyseal forearm fractures. Therefore, closed reduction maneuvers for these injuries are not described below. However, two common injuries about the elbow and forearm that are frequently treated nonsurgically are the simple elbow dislocation and the nightstick ulnar shaft fracture.

Elbow Dislocation

Indication

Elbow dislocations with and without fractures should be promptly reduced. Most simple elbow dislocations can be treated nonsurgically with closed reduction, followed by a short period of immobilization. After initial closed reduction, many complex elbow dislocations will require surgical treatment to restore stability and/or to reestablish articular congruency.

Description of Procedure

For all techniques, patient comfort is paramount. We routinely perform closed reduction after an intraarticular elbow injection of 5 cc of 1% lidocaine. Alternatively, conscious sedation can be used to provide anesthesia for reduction. All techniques start with correction of medial/lateral displacement, followed by traction and flexion.

SUPINE TECHNIQUE

- Position the patient supine, with the bed height adjusted to place the elbow at the level of your waist. With the elbow extended, stabilize the arm while using your other hand to manipulate the proximal forearm to correct any medial/lateral displacement. This will allow the trochlea and ulna to align and allow reduction of the trochlea in the next step of the procedure (Fig. 3-5).

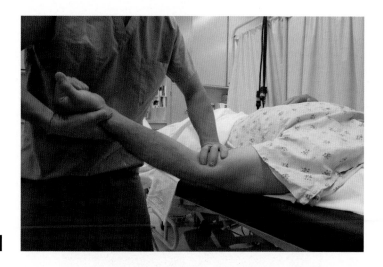

FIGURE
3-5

■ With an assistant providing countertraction, pull gentle longitudinal traction with the elbow extended. Place the thumb of your contralateral hand on the tip of the olecranon and grasp the anterior humerus to provide counterpressure. Now, use your thumb to place a firm anterior force on the olecranon. As the elbow is slowly flexed, the reduction occurs, often with a palpable clunk (Fig. 3-6).

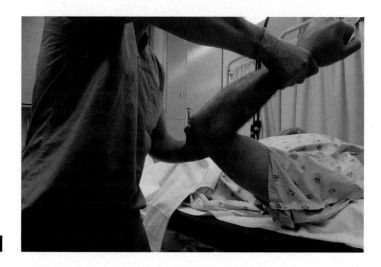

FIGURE
3-6

■ Perform a stability examination.
■ Place the elbow at 90° of flexion and neutral rotation in a long-arm posterior splint.

PRONE TECHNIQUE

■ The patient is placed prone, with the arm hanging over the side of the bed.
■ Correct any medial/lateral displacement as described above.

■ An assistant pulls longitudinal traction. Cup the elbow with both thumbs on the tip of the olecranon and digits in the antecubital fossa. As your assistant flexes the elbow, place firm anterior force on the olecranon. Reduction will occur with a palpable clunk (Fig. 3-7).

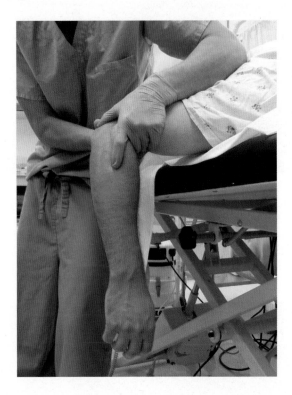

FIGURE
3-7

■ Perform a stability examination, and apply a splint as described above.

Tips and Other Considerations

■ To anesthetize the elbow using an intraarticular injection, use the same technique as described above. However, you will have a larger area to aim for since the joint is dislocated, opening up a wide intraarticular space. Aspiration of the hematoma confirms intraarticular needle placement and assists with pain relief.

■ After a successful reduction, it is paramount to perform a stability examination to guide further treatment. We prefer to bring the elbow through its range of motion while observing the lateral image under live minifluoroscopy. Record the degree of extension at which the elbow starts to subluxate. Next, an anteroposterior image is viewed while providing gentle varus and valgus stress with the elbow at 30° of flexion. Alternatively, the stability examination can be easily done clinically without fluoroscopy.

■ The majority of patients with simple elbow dislocations are sufficiently stable to start early range of motion at 3 to 5 days postreduction. To prevent stiffness, these patients should be given early follow-up appointments.

Ulnar Shaft Fracture: "Nightstick Fracture"

Indication

Closed treatment is indicated for ulnar shaft fractures which are minimally displaced. Although closed reduction can provide small corrections for fractures that are borderline, it should not be used for definitive treatment in significantly displaced or angulated fractures. Additionally, the elbow should be closely inspected for radial head fracture/dislocation to rule out a Monteggia injury.

Tolerances

<50% translation and <10° angulation.

Description of Procedure

- Place the patient supine, with the arm draped over the chest.
- A hematoma block may be used for anesthesia during reduction. After a sterile preparation at the fracture site, use a 22G needle to pierce the skin over the subcutaneous border of the ulna at the fracture site. When the needle enters the fracture site, aspirate the hematoma confirming accurate placement and inject 5 cc of 1% lidocaine.
- Typically, the fracture is most stable in supination; however, we recommend only moderate (≤45°) supination because the patient will quickly lose pronation if splinted in full supination.
- A long-arm cast is placed to hold the arm in this position. A flat mold over the dorsoulnar border of the forearm is used to straighten the ulna. To achieve this, we rub a flat palm firmly over this surface. Alternatively, a flat object can be used to mold the cast.

PEDIATRIC CONSIDERATIONS—CLOSED ELBOW REDUCTIONS

Supracondylar Humerus Fractures

Indication

Nondisplaced fractures are treated without manipulation by immobilization in a long-arm cast.

Closed reduction and splinting/casting may be indicated for displaced supracondylar humerus fractures in children with an intact posterior cortex (Fig. 3-8).

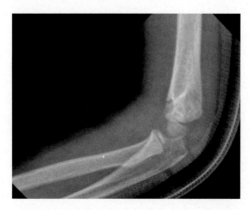

FIGURE
3-8

Widely displaced fractures, defined by lack of posterior cortical contact, should have definitive surgical repair. We do not routinely perform a provisional closed reduction of widely displaced fractures unless there is skin compromise or neurovascular injury. In the absence of these soft tissue injuries, the elbow is splinted in a position of comfort prior to operative treatment (Fig. 3-9).

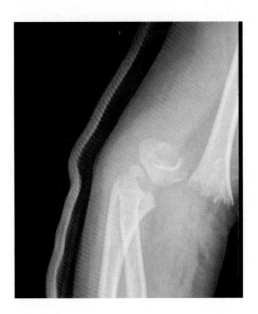

FIGURE

3-9

Tolerances

The anterior humeral line should pass through the middle one-third of the ossification center of the capitellum (Fig. 3-10). If it passes posterior to this ossification center, then a residual extension deformity exists. On the AP image, the shaft/physeal (Baumann) angle should be within 5° of the contralateral elbow (average is 85° to 89°) (Fig. 3-11).

Description of Procedure

- Although flexion type supracondylar humerus fractures exist, here we describe the treatment of the much more common (>95%) extension type fracture.
- We prefer conscious sedation for anesthesia when manipulating most pediatric fractures. Position the patient supine, with the affected shoulder at the edge of the bed.
- The first step is gentle traction with the arm in extension to align the fracture. Grasp the upper arm with your outside hand and the forearm with your inside hand and pull moderate traction. This step often corrects varus/valgus angulation and malrotation due to tension on the soft tissue envelop. Subtle changes in alignment are made in extension by holding the arm stable and adjusting the forearm (Fig. 3-12).
- Slide the hand that is grasping the arm down to the elbow and place your thumb over the tip of the olecranon. Now flex the elbow while placing a firm anterior force on the olecranon to reduce the extension deformity (Fig. 3-13). As you flex the elbow, pronate the

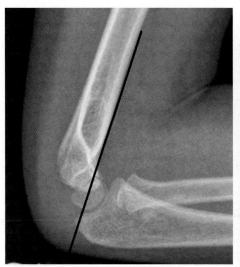

FIGURE
3-10

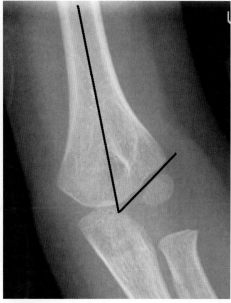

FIGURE
3-11

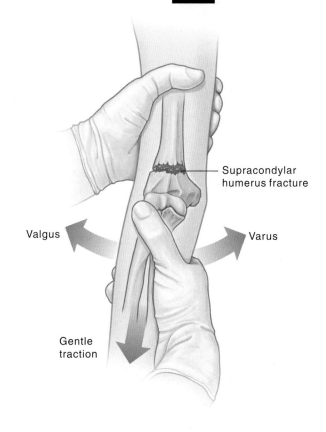

Supracondylar
humerus fracture

Valgus

Varus

Gentle
traction

FIGURE
3-12

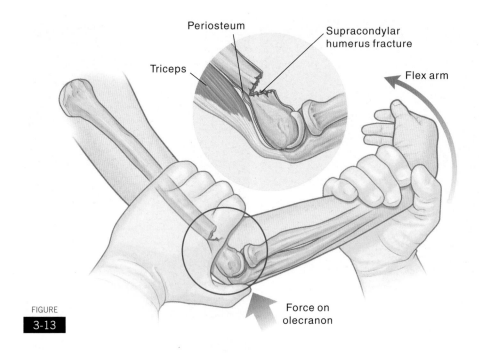

Periosteum

Supracondylar
humerus fracture

Triceps

Flex arm

FIGURE
3-13

Force on
olecranon

forearm to lock the reduction (most fractures are more stable in pronation). This reduction maneuver relies on both an intact posterior periosteum and the triceps as a tension band (Fig. 3-14).

■ Slide your hand from the tip of the olecranon back up to the arm to allow the cast technician to place a long-arm cast with the elbow at 90° and the forearm in pronation. Once the cast is placed, put a mold over the posterior elbow to maintain the correction of the extension deformity.

Tips and Other Considerations

■ If the vascular exam is abnormal, then attempt a closed reduction and reevaluate the vascular status.

■ Pronation of the forearm is used to tighten the medial hinge, providing correction of medial translation and varus. Supination is the opposite, correcting lateral translation and valgus deformities.

■ Greater than 90° of elbow flexion is often required to achieve the reduction, but the elbow should not be immobilized in >90° of flexion. If >90° of elbow flexion is required to maintain the reduction, then nonoperative treatment is abandoned. The arm is splinted in a position of comfort in the interim.

Lateral Condyle Fracture

We do not perform closed reduction and splinting/casting of lateral condyle fractures. If the fragment is displaced <2 mm, we place a long-arm cast in 60° to 90° flexion with the forearm in neutral rotation. If the fracture is ≥2 mm displaced, we proceed with surgical

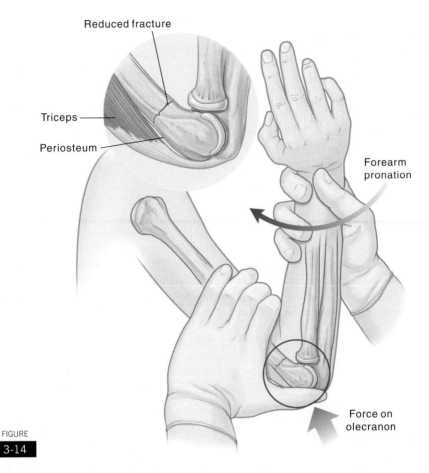

Reduced fracture

Triceps

Periosteum

Forearm pronation

Force on olecranon

FIGURE
3-14

treatment. Any patient with a lateral condyle fracture that is treated nonsurgically should follow up in less than 1 week for repeat x-rays, as these fractures are known to displace in the cast.

Incarcerated Medial Epicondyle

Indication

Medial epicondyle fractures are the most common fracture in the setting of a pediatric elbow dislocation. During an elbow dislocation, the medial epicondyle is avulsed and can become incarcerated in the elbow joint. An attempt should be made to remove the entrapped fragment prior to reduction of the elbow dislocation.

Description of Procedure

- Conscious sedation is recommended. Place the patient supine.
- To extract the medial epicondyle, place a valgus load on the elbow while simultaneously maximally supinating the forearm and dorsiflexing the wrist and digits.

- Once the fragment is extracted, proceed with closed reduction of the elbow dislocation as described above for adults.
- Place the elbow in a long-arm posterior splint at 90° flexion.

Tips and Other Considerations

- If you fail to extract the fragment prior to reduction, then try reducing the elbow first, which occasionally pushes the fragment out of the joint.
- The patient should follow up for repeat x-rays to confirm stability and start early (3 to 7 days) range of motion.

Radial Head/Neck Fracture

Indication

The radial neck can remodel when minimal angulation is present. A successful closed reduction is desired, because operative treatment frequently results in elbow stiffness.

For all techniques, the patient is supine, with the affected shoulder at the edge of the bed. Conscious sedation is our preferred mechanism of anesthesia. After a reduction has been achieved, splint or cast the elbow at 90° and moderate to full pronation. A posterolaterally based mold can help maintain the reduction.

Tolerances

- <30° angulation: no manipulation.
- 30° to 60° angulation: closed reduction attempt.
- >60° angulation: consider primary operative treatment.

Description of Procedure

PATTERSON TECHNIQUE[1]

- An assistant grasps the upper arm for countertraction and to provide a medial post at the elbow for varus force.
- With the elbow extended and supinated, grasp the patient's forearm and provide traction and a firm varus moment at the elbow.
- To complete the reduction, take the thumb of your other hand and push the radial head medially.

JEFFREY TECHNIQUE (AUTHOR'S PREFERRED TECHNIQUE)[2]

- This method is similar to Patterson technique. Your assistant holds the patient's arm in the same manner as above.
- Using palpation directly lateral to the radial head or an AP fluoroscopic image, pronate and supinate the patient's forearm so that the radial head is most prominent directly lateral. This places the plane of maximal angulation so that a direct lateral force provides the most effective reduction (Fig. 3-15).
- With the elbow extended and the forearm rotated according to the previous step, provide traction and varus forces.
- To complete the reduction, place the thumb of your opposite hand directly laterally over the maximum prominence and firmly push the radial medially to complete the reduction.

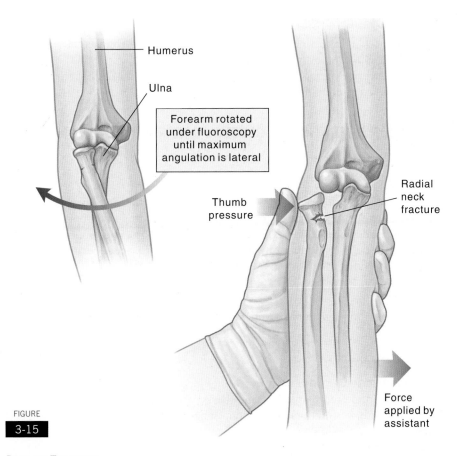

Humerus

Ulna

Forearm rotated under fluoroscopy until maximum angulation is lateral

Thumb pressure

Radial neck fracture

Force applied by assistant

FIGURE
3-15

BANDAGE TECHNIQUE

■ With elbow extended, wrap an Esmarch bandage from the wrist to well above the elbow in a distal to proximal direction. The soft tissue tension may reduce the radial neck fracture.

■ In our experience, this technique is less effective and should only be used in fractures that are minimally angulated. Conscious sedation is still required, as most children do not tolerate this procedure well.

Radial Head Subluxation: "Nursemaid's Elbow"

Indication

All patients with radial head subluxation should undergo closed reduction.

Description of Procedure

■ No anesthesia is required. Place your thumb over the radial head and provide gentle posteromedial-directed pressure. With the elbow in full extension, gently supinate the forearm. Complete the reduction by fully flexing the elbow. The radial head will reduce with a palpable clunk.

■ No immobilization is necessary. The child should resume immediate use of the extremity.

Tips and Other Considerations

- If you experience difficulty with reduction, then make sure that you flex the elbow >90° as this is required in a minority of children.
- Rarely this maneuver will fail to reduce the radial head. In this case, hyperpronate the forearm in a flexed position to achieve a reduction.

PEDIATRIC CONSIDERATIONS—CLOSED FOREARM REDUCTIONS

Radial and Ulnar Shaft Fractures

Indication

The treatment of the pediatric both-bone forearm fracture depends on the fracture characteristics and the ability of the child to remodel. The most important fracture characteristics include the degree of angular and rotational deformity. The most important patient characteristic is the patient's age. It is our policy to reduce all displaced pediatric combined radius and ulna fractures.

Tolerances

- ≤10 years old: <15° of angulation, bayonet apposition accepted.
- >10 years old: <10° angulation.

Description of Procedure

- Position the child supine, with the affected shoulder at the edge of the bed. Conscious sedation is our preferred method of anesthesia. The steps of the reduction are restoration of length, restoration of rotational alignment, and restoration of angular alignment.
- Restoration of length.
  - Longitudinal traction is applied, which often allows some level of self-correction of rotational malalignment. In cases of complete displacement, traction to reestablish length will facilitate later angular correction (Fig. 3-16).
  - In cases of complete displacement with overriding fracture ends, inline traction, no matter how vigorous, often fails to achieve apposed bone ends. To achieve apposition

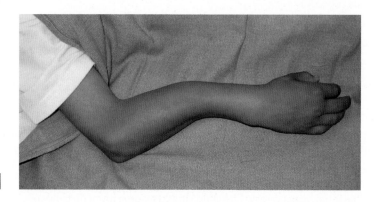

FIGURE
3-16

of the fracture ends, first recreate the injury mechanism. This requires exaggeration of the angular deformity followed by traction.

- ▪ Often a thumb proximal to the fracture on the concave side of the deformity is useful to push the overriding fracture end to the correct position.
- ▪ Restoration of rotation.
  - ▪ The rotational alignment of the forearm is now addressed. In general, if the fracture of the radius is proximal to the insertion of the pronator teres, then the forearm should be immobilized in supination. When the radius fracture is distal to the pronator teres insertion, we generally immobilize in neutral rotation. For distal combined radial and ulnar fractures, the forearm is often most stable in neutral rotation to pronation.
- ▪ Restoration of angulation.
  - ▪ Next reduce angular deformity. Typically, children have an intact periosteal hinge on the concave side of the fracture. Maintain traction, while applying a 3- or 4-point bending force. Using either your palm or digits as a fulcrum, straighten the forearm (Figs. 3-17 and 3-18).

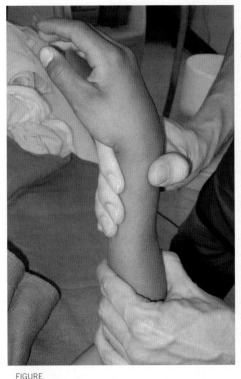

FIGURE
3-17

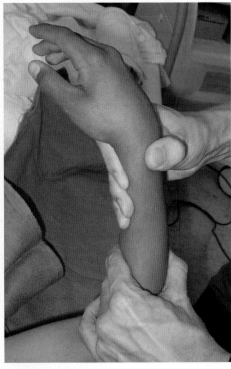

FIGURE
3-18

- ▪ An assistant applies a long-arm cast. To maintain the reduction, two important molds must be placed. An interosseous mold is placed by taking the palms of both hands and gently squeezing the forearm at the level of the fracture. This increases the interosseous width and helps restore the radial bow, which improves forearm rotation. Additionally, the interosseous mold creates an oval cast, which has been shown to be more effective than a cylindrical cast (Fig. 3-19).

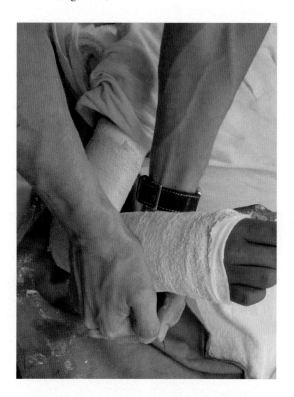

FIGURE
3-19

- A 3-point mold is now placed to maintain the angular correction. There are multiple methods to place this mold: (1) Place one hand at the apex of the fracture and the other hand on the opposite side of the distal fragment. Place your knee on the side opposite to the apex over the proximal fragment and provide a bending moment. (2) Place the patients forearm over your knee with the apex side down. Provide a bending moment over your knee.
- For all fractures proximal to the distal radial metaphysis, your cast or splint must control forearm rotation. This can be achieved with a sugar-tong splint or a long-arm cast, but short-arm casts or splints cannot be used in these fractures.

Tips and Other Considerations

- The rules regarding rotation apply in most cases. However, a mini c-arm is useful to adjust the rotational alignment on a case-by-case basis.
- Greenstick fractures: Often these fractures will drift back to their initial angulation during follow-up visits. Therefore, we will accentuate the reduction to overcorrect the angular deformity. Occasionally, this results in completion of the fracture, which usually poses no issue. However, the clinician should be aware that after the completion of a greenstick

fracture, translation and rotational deformity may occur, which is occasionally challenging to correct.

■ Plastic deformity: Occasionally, either the radius or ulna will not overtly fracture but become plastically deformed. In these cases, alert the physician who is performing conscious sedation that the procedure will take longer than usual. Plastic deformity invariably takes a significant amount of force to reduce. Although a large amount of force will be required, it must be applied gradually to prevent overt fracture of the bone. If the bone fractures prior to correction of the deformity, then all hope is lost for correction of the bow.

■ Swelling: We prefer to place all children in a cast since it is easier to maintain the reduction and decreases the risk of redisplacement during the change to a cast in clinic. If a reduction is performed, then we always valve the cast. In the case of mild swelling, univalving the cast is sufficient. When swelling is more severe, we bivalve the cast, and in the most severe of cases, section the Webril as well. We try to cut the cast in a way to prevent motion in the plane of maximal fracture angulation. For instance, if the fracture was dorsally displaced, then the cast is bivalved on the dorsal and volar surfaces to allow expansion radially/ulnarly but not dorsally/volarly.

Monteggia Fracture/Dislocation

Indication

A Monteggia fracture classically involves a proximal ulna fracture combined with dislocation of the radial head. All Monteggia fracture/dislocations should be identified and reduced. Anytime a child presents with an isolated ulna fracture, a Monteggia injury should be assumed until proven otherwise. High-quality elbow radiographs are necessary to evaluate the elbow.

Description of Procedure

■ Place the child supine, with the shoulder at the edge of the bed. Conscious sedation is administered. Most commonly in children, the ulna is displaced apex anterior, and the radial head is dislocated anteriorly.

■ The first step in reducing the Monteggia injury is anatomic correction of the ulna. During this maneuver, the radial head often self-reduces.

■ The forearm is supinated, and an assistant stabilizes the arm. Place your palm at the apex of the ulna fracture on the volar aspect of the forearm. Use your contralateral hand to grasp the dorsal aspect of the distal forearm. Provide a strong force to correct the apex anterior ulnar deformity.

■ Often, the radial head will reduce after this maneuver. If it is still subluxated or dislocated, then reassess the ulnar alignment. Most commonly, the ulna is nonanatomic. If the ulna is anatomic but the radial head is still dislocated, then maximally supinate the forearm and place firm pressure over the lateral aspect of the radial head.

■ A long-arm cast is placed with the forearm supinated and the elbow at 90°.

■ The patient will require close follow-up for early detection of radial head instability.

Tips and Other Considerations

■ Beware of the ulna that is plastically deformed. Achieving an anatomic reduction in this case is difficult and requires significant force often necessitating general anesthesia.

Galeazzi Fracture/Dislocation

Indication

A Galeazzi fracture/dislocation involves fracture of the radial shaft, typically at the junction of the middle and distal one-thirds, and dislocation of the distal radioulnar joint. Unlike adults, in children, Galeazzi fractures are often successfully treated with closed reduction and cast immobilization.

Description of Procedure

- Galeazzi fractures are notoriously difficult to reduce, as it is often difficult to reestablish proper length of the radius when the ulna is intact. For this reason, deep conscious sedation is necessary. Move the child so that their shoulder is at the edge of the bed.
- A large amount of traction is often necessary to achieve proper radial length. It is useful to have an assistant pull countertraction. As in combined radius and ulna fractures, exaggeration of the deformity may be required to achieve radial length.
- Once radial length is achieved, then angular correction of the radius is achieved, with 3-point bending. As with other forearm fractures, while an assistant stabilizes the arm, use one hand at the apex of the fracture and the other on the wrist to correct angulation.
- In the more common case of a dorsally displaced distal radioulnar joint dislocation, immobilize the forearm in near-full supination. In the less commonly encountered volar distal radioulnar joint dislocation, immobilize the forearm in near-full pronation.
- Once a long-arm cast is applied, place similar molds as a both-bone forearm fracture. First, perform an interosseous mold, followed by a 3-point bending mold.

Tips and Other Considerations

- An assistant and complete patient relaxation are crucial to allow a large amount of traction to be generated.
- If you are unsure about ulnar variance (relative heights of ulna and radius at the wrist) or reduction of the distal radioulnar joint, then obtain a fluoroscopic image of the uninjured wrist. The ulnar variance can be measured by an AP image of the wrist. The distal radioulnar joint reduction can be compared to the lateral of the uninjured wrist to ensure that no dorsal or volar subluxation exists.

PROCEDURE FOR COMPARTMENT PRESSURE MEASUREMENT IN THE FOREARM

Indication

Compartment syndrome occurs when the pressure within the fascial compartment exceeds capillary pressure, leading to tissue ischemia. It is an orthopaedic emergency and requires emergent fasciotomy. The use of compartment pressure measurement in the diagnosis of compartment syndrome is controversial. Because false negatives and false positives can occur, pressure measurements can fluctuate with time and proximity to the traumatized tissue, and the pressure that defines compartment syndrome is unknown, we prefer to make the diagnosis on the basis of clinical examination when possible. Compartment pressure measurement is utilized when the patient is intoxicated, obtunded, or otherwise incapable of cooperating with an examination. When performed, we define compartment syndrome when the compartment pressure is within 30 mm Hg of the patient's diastolic blood pressure.

Description of Procedure

- The forearm contains three compartments: volar, dorsal, and mobile wad (Fig. 3-20).
- Position the patient supine.
- Prepare a wide area of the skin with antibacterial solution.
- *Optional:* Mark the entry site with a marking pen. Perform this step prior to application of antibacterial solution if a nonsterile pen is used.
- Three entry sites are required to access the compartments of the forearm:
  - Volar compartment: Unlike the other forearm compartments, major nerves and arteries are in close proximity to the insertion site. The entry site is located on the volar aspect of the forearm immediately ulnar to the palmaris longus. This insertion site avoids the median and ulnar nerves as well as the radial and ulnar nerves. In general, we measure the pressure at the junction of the middle and proximal forearm. The needle insertion depth is 1 to 2 cm (Fig. 3-21).
  - Dorsal compartment: The entry site is 1 fingerbreadth radial to the palpable ulna on the dorsum of the forearm. In general, we measure the pressure at the junction of the middle and proximal forearm. The needle insertion depth is 1 to 2 cm (Fig. 3-22).
  - Mobile wad: The needle insertion point is the most radial aspect of the proximal forearm. Palpate the lateral column of the humerus. The insertion site is the fleshy mass distal and volar to the lateral epicondyle. The needle insertion depth is 2 cm (Fig. 3-23).

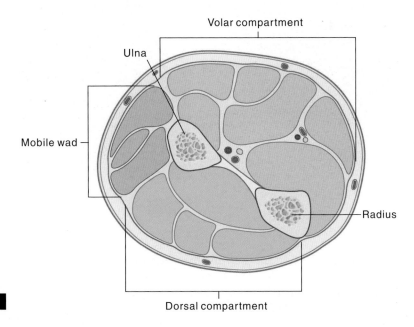

FIGURE
3-20

Volar compartment

Ulna

Mobile wad

Radius

Dorsal compartment

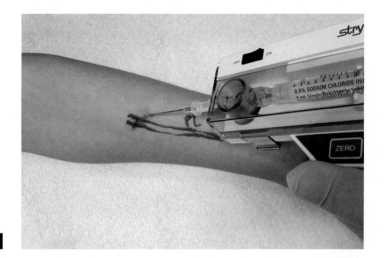

FIGURE
3-21

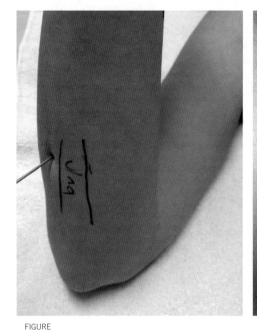

FIGURE
3-22

FIGURE
3-23

- *Optional:* Anesthetize the skin overlying the planned entry site with 2 to 3 ml of local anesthetic.
- Assemble the intracompartmental-pressure-measuring device according to the manufacturer's specifications (Fig. 3-24).

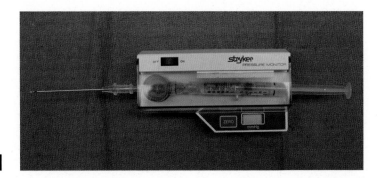

FIGURE
3-24

■ Alternatively, an arterial line system with high-pressure tubing and a wick or slit catheter can be used (Fig. 3-25). The least desirable needle is a standard hypodermic needle because the opening has a small surface area, and is easily clogged.

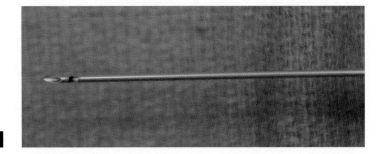

FIGURE
3-25

■ Hold the needle/pressure transducer at the level of the entry site and at the angle of insertion. Zero the system and perform three measurements per compartment.

Tips and Other Considerations

■ To determine the proper insertion depth, use a sterile marking pen to place 1- and 2-cm hash marks on the needle.
■ If you are unsure that the needle is subfascial, then you can flex and extend the patient's fingers and wrist. The pressure wave should cause fluctuations in the pressure readings.
■ Have an assistant write down the pressure measurements as you call them out.

REFERENCES

1. Patterson RF. Treatment of displaced transverse fractures of the neck of the radius in children. *J Bone Joint Surg*. 1934;16:696–698.
2. Jeffrey CC. Fractures of the head of the radius in children. *J Bone Joint Surg Br*. 1950;32:314–324.

The Wrist and Hand

INJECTIONS AND ASPIRATIONS

Distal Radius Hematoma Block

Indication

A hematoma block is used to anesthetize the distal radius for closed reduction maneuvers.

Description of Procedure

- Position the patient either sitting with the wrist resting on a mayo stand or supine (our preference) with the wrist comfortably by the side.
- Prepare the overlying skin with alcohol, Betadine, or chlorhexidine gluconate (our preference).
- Palpate the bony landmarks of the wrist noting the position of the radial and ulnar styloids and the dorsal fracture step-off. The entry site is on the dorsal of the wrist directly central on the radius at the level of the fracture.
- *Optional:* The overlying skin is anesthetized with 2 to 3 cc of 1% lidocaine without epinephrine using a 25G to 30G needle. The use of local anesthetic is debatable. Some physicians feel it is not helpful because only the skin will be anesthetized, and a second injection is required. We do not routinely use local anesthetic prior to skin penetration. However, the needle should penetrate the skin quickly to minimize pain.
- Using a 5 to 10 cc syringe with a 22G needle pierce the skin and advance the needle down to the fracture site. It is critical that the needle enter the fracture. If intact bone is felt, then walk the needle distally and proximally until it falls into the fracture.
- Once the needle is in the fracture site, aspirate hematoma to confirm placement. A rush of blood will be seen. Now inject ≤5 cc of 1% lidocaine (Fig. 4-1).

Tips and Other Considerations

- For the dorsally displaced fracture, always err on inserting the needle more proximal. This allows the needle to angle distally into the fracture site. If you insert the needle even the slightest bit distal to the fracture site, it is impossible to insert the needle into the fracture (Fig. 4-2).
- A hematoma block is only effective for acute fractures. In our experience, the best results are obtained in fractures that are ≤3 days old. With each successive day, the efficacy of the block is reduced.
- We have found that it takes at least 5 to 10 minutes for the block to work. This delayed effect is different from the near immediate effectiveness of lidocaine when infiltrated in the skin.

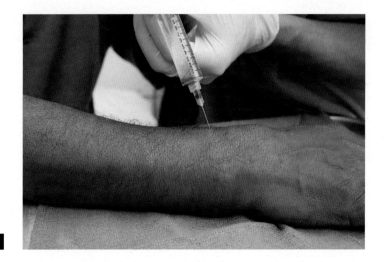

FIGURE
4-1

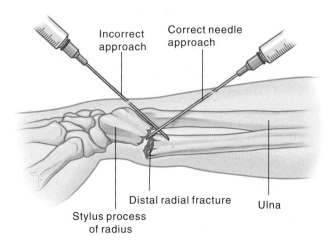

FIGURE
4-2

Incorrect approach

Correct needle approach

Distal radial fracture

Ulna

Stylus process of radius

■ Use caution when injecting >5 mL of lidocaine since it may increase carpal tunnel pressure.

■ We do not recommend performing hematoma blocks on the volar side of the wrist.

Intra-articular Wrist Injection / Aspiration

Indication

Accurate placement of a needle into the wrist joint can be useful to obtain synovial fluid for analysis in the diagnosis of septic arthritis and inflammatory arthritides. It can also be used to administer therapeutic agents or for anesthesia during the reduction of perilunate injuries.

Description of Procedure

- The patient can be either seated or supine. The dorsum of the wrist is sterilely prepped.
- Palpate Lister tubercle on the dorsum of the wrist. The radiocarpal joint line can be palpated as a depression just distal to Lister tubercle (Fig. 4-3).
- The wrist joint has multiple compartments and depending on the pathology, you may wish to place the needle in a particular area.
    - If the radiocarpal joint is desired, then position the wrist in neutral extension. Pierce the skin with a 22G to 25G needle just distal to the joint line on the dorsum of the wrist. Angle the needle 10° to 15° proximally to clear the proximal pole of the scaphoid and enter the joint (Fig. 4-4).

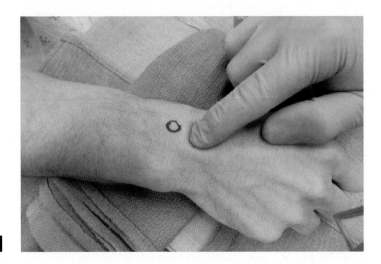

FIGURE
4-3

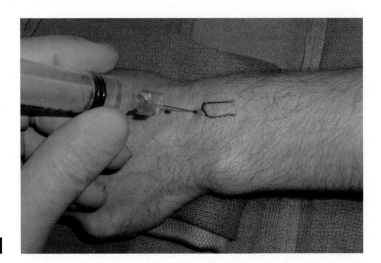

FIGURE
4-4

■ If the midcarpal joint is desired, then place the wrist in a small amount of flexion (approximately 10°). Pierce the skin 1.5 cm distal to Lister tubercle (1 cm distal to your radiocarpal entry point). Your needle will enter the wrist between the capitate and the proximal carpal row (proximal scaphoid or lunate) (Fig. 4-5).

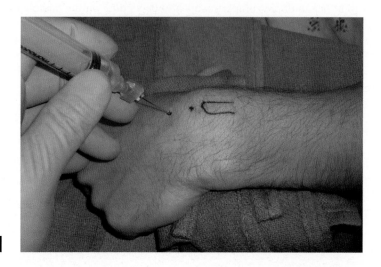

FIGURE
4-5

Tips and Other Considerations

■ Because the wrist is a small joint, if you encounter difficulty entering the joint, then place the patient in finger traps with 10 lb of traction (alternatively an assistant can pull traction). This opens the joint spaces, making placement easier.
■ In cases of trauma and infection, the dorsum of the wrist is often massively swollen. In these cases, use of fluoroscopy to mark your entry site is required.

Carpal Tunnel Injection

Indication

A carpal tunnel injection may be used in the nonsurgical treatment of chronic carpel tunnel syndrome. In this scenario, the injection is therapeutic and provides prognostic information regarding pain relief after carpel tunnel release. An aspiration can be performed in the rare case in which a suppurative carpel tunnel syndrome is suspected.

Description of Procedure

■ The patient can be either supine or seated with the volar aspect of the wrist exposed.
■ Determine the location of the palmaris longus tendon (if present) by having the patient press the pads of the thumb and small finger together while simultaneously flexing the wrist 30°. The palmaris longus typically lies directly over the median nerve (Fig. 4-6).
■ The entry point is at the distal wrist crease just ulnar to the palmaris longus. Using a 25G needle pierce the skin at this point with the needle angled distally 45° to the skin. Often you will feel the needle pierce the transverse carpal ligament with a tactile "pop" (Fig. 4-7).

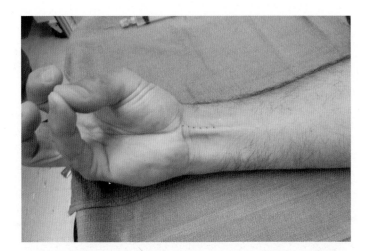

FIGURE
4-6

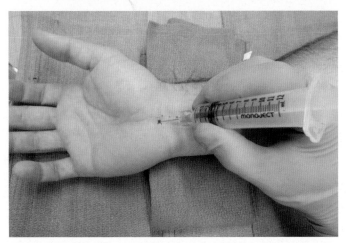

FIGURE
4-7

- Aspirate (if suppurative carpal tunnel syndrome is suspected) or inject 2 cc of 1% lido-caine mixed with 1 cc of triamcinolone (40 mg/mL). If resistance is felt or if the patient experiences paresthesias, the needle should be removed to the level of the skin and redirected more ulnarly.

First Dorsal Compartment Injection

Indication

A corticosteroid injection into the first dorsal compartment is used in the nonsurgical treatment of de Quervain disease.

Description of Procedure

- The wrist is ulnarly deviated slightly (10° to 15°). *Optional:* A small bump, which maintains the wrist in slight ulnar deviation, is fashioned for the patient to rest their hand on (Fig. 4-8).

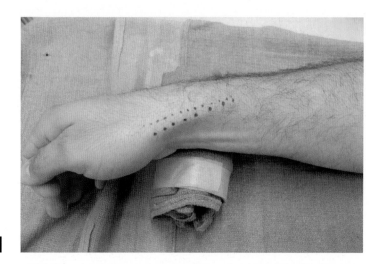

FIGURE
4-8

- Have the patient give a "thumbs up" sign. The extensor pollicis longus and abductor pollicis brevis tendons can be seen and palpated in the first dorsal compartment. These tendons are most easily felt just distally to the radial styloid. Follow them proximally to the level of the radial styloid and, mark this point (Fig. 4-9).
- With the thumb relaxed, pierce the skin with a 25G needle at the marked point. The needle should enter the skin at a 45° angle with the tip pointing distally. To avoid injection directly into a tendon slowly move the thumb; the needle should remain in the same position (Fig. 4-10).
- Inject 1 cc of 1% lidocaine and 1 cc of triamcinolone (40 mg/mL). The fluid should flow easily; if resistance is met either the needle is in a tendon or not in the correct compartment. As you inject, a visual sign that the needle position is accurate is the expansion of first dorsal compartment distally.

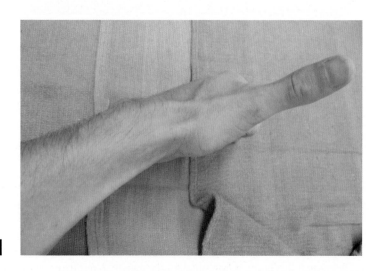

FIGURE
4-9

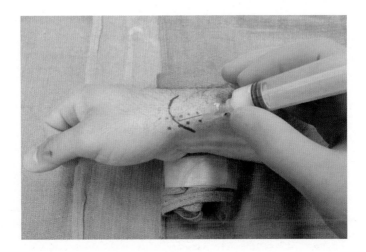

FIGURE
4-10

Base of Thumb Carpometacarpal Joint Injection

Indication

The most common indication for this injection is administration of therapeutics for base of the thumb arthritis. It can also be used to infiltrate lidocaine for pain relief during the reduction of Bennett fractures of the thumb.

Description of Procedure

- Locate the apex of the anatomic snuffbox on the dorsoradial side of the hand. The entry site is near the apex of the snuffbox (Fig. 4-11).
- Passively flex and extend the thumb to palpate the joint line. Once the joint line is located, it is easiest to enter with the thumb in flexion.
- Pierce the skin and joint capsule at a perpendicular angle and administer 0.5 cc of 1% lidocaine and 0.5 cc of triamcinolone (40 mg/mL) for the treatment of arthritis or 1 cc of 1% lidocaine for anesthesia during reduction maneuvers (Fig. 4-12).

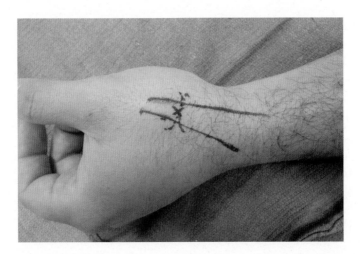

FIGURE
4-11

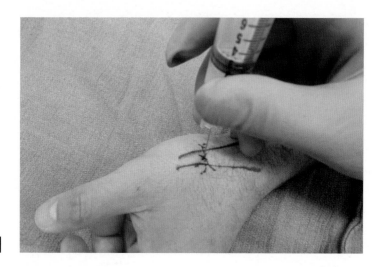

FIGURE
4-12

Tips and Other Considerations

- This is a small joint, therefore it is helpful to have an assistant pull traction on the thumb to open the joint space or use a single finger trap (5 lb).
- A 25G needle is helpful to enter this small joint.

Digital Nerve Block

Indication

A digital nerve block is used to anesthetize the digit for reductions or procedures. A digital nerve block provides adequate anesthesia for reductions and procedures distal to the mid-point of the proximal phalanx. It is less reliable for work around the base of the digit.

Description of Procedure

STANDARD DIGITAL NERVE BLOCK

- At the level of the webspace, the digital nerves are located relatively volar, just at the periphery of the flexor tendon sheath. There exist smaller dorsal nerve branches which run along the dorsal aspect of the digit.
- Because the nerves are located volarly, we recommend a volar approach to the nerve in most cases, however if you only plan to work on the dorsal aspect of the digit a dorsal approach can be used.
- Position the hand with the palm up and the digits extended. Palpate the flexor tendon sheath; the needle is inserted centrally over the tendon sheath.
- Using a 25 guage needle, pierce the skin of the centrally over the metacarpophalangeal (MCP) joint. Angle the needle 30° toward the webspace, and inject 0.5 mL 1% lidocaine without epinephrine. Withdraw enough to redirect but not out of the skin. Redirect the needle 30° to the opposite webspace. Inject an addition 0.5 cc to anesthetize the other digital nerve (Figs. 4-13 and 4-14).

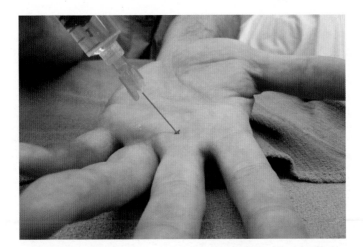

FIGURE
4-13

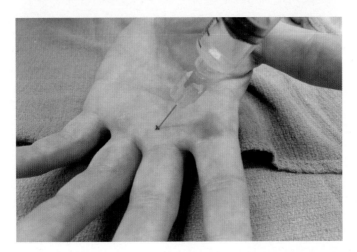

FIGURE
4-14

FLEXOR TENDON SHEATH BLOCK

■ Position the hand with the volar aspect up. Palpate the flexor tendon sheath of the digit of interest. The entry site of the injection is the same as the standard digital nerve block, centrally over the sheath at the level of the MCP joint, however the direction of the needle is different.

■ Using a 25G needle, pierce the skin at this point, and advance the needle perpendicular to the skin. The needle will enter the flexor tendon sheath and should be advanced until the firm endpoint of the volar plate is felt.

■ Withdraw the needle 1 to 2 mm and inject 2 to 3 cc 1% lidocaine. There should be minimal resistance to the injection if correctly placed. There are two ways to confirm correct placement: (1) Palpate the flexor tendon sheath distally over the proximal phalanx, and as you inject you should be able to feel a pressure wave. (2) If the needle is correctly placed as you inject, the patient will feel a rush of fluid up the digit (Figs. 4-15 and 4-16).

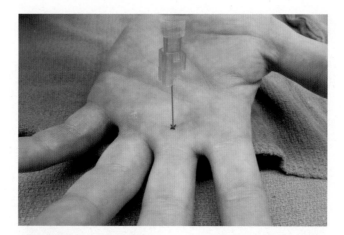

FIGURE
4-15

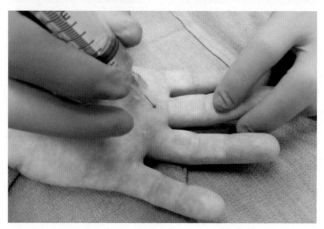

FIGURE
4-16

Tips and Other Considerations

- We prefer to use a flexor tendon sheath block for all of our digital blocks. It provides excellent anesthesia of the digit with a single needle stick. We have had no failures with this technique even when working on the dorsum of the digit.
- To perform a trigger finger injection, use the same technique as the flexor tendon sheath block, but inject 1 cc of 1% lidocaine mixed with 1 cc of triamcinolone (40 mg/mL).

CLOSED REDUCTIONS

Distal Radius Fracture

Indication

Closed reduction of a distal radius fracture is indicated in the initial management of displaced distal radius fractures. It should be urgently performed in the setting of median nerve dysfunction prior to surgical management. In a select group of patients, closed reduction and immobilization may be used for definitive treatment of a distal radius fracture.

We routinely perform manipulation of distal radius fractures using a hematoma block (see above) for anesthesia. The methods described are for the common dorsal displaced distal radius fracture (e.g., Colles fracture). Volarly angulated fractures (e.g., Smith fractures) are more difficult to treat nonoperatively and shear fractures (e.g., Barton fractures) are usually impossible to treat nonoperatively.

Tolerances

- Radial shortening < 3 mm.
- Radial inclination > 15°.
- Dorsal tilt < 10°.
- Ulnar variance within 2 mm of uninjured side.

Description of Procedure

A variety of techniques can be used to reduce the distal radius. The basic principle is to provide longitudinal traction while recreating the injury mechanism to realign the radius. The differences between techniques only involve the method of traction applied depending on the level of patient comfort and number of assistants available. The technique is similar in children and adults, and any differences are mentioned below.

STANDARD TECHNIQUE

- After performing a hematoma block, position the patient supine with the ipsilateral shoulder at the edge of the bed. The elbow should be flexed to relax many of the forearm muscles.
- An assistant grasps the arm to provide countertraction. Grasp the patient's hand firmly around the thumb using the same side as that of the patient's injured side (if the patient's right wrist is fractured then use your right hand). Firmly pull toward the ceiling to provide traction (Fig. 4-17).

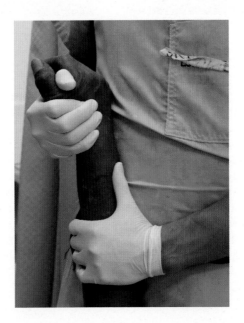

FIGURE
4-17

- Place your contralateral hand dorsally just proximal to the fracture site to provide a fulcrum. As you continue to pull traction hyperextend the wrist, recreating the injury mechanism (Fig. 4-18).
- To complete the reduction, slide your thumb distally over the distal fragment, and provide a firm anterior and distal force while simultaneously flexing, ulnar deviating, and pronating the wrist (Fig. 4-19).

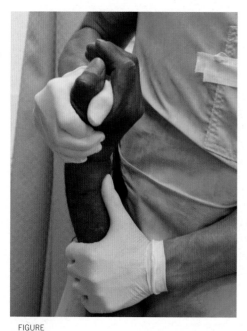

FIGURE
4-18

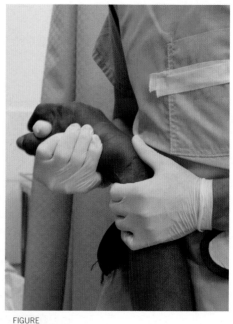

FIGURE
4-19

- It is important to translate the distal fragment volarly to correct dorsal displacement prior to flexing the fragment. If the fragment is prematurely flexed, it is impossible to translate and some stability is lost (Fig. 4-20).
- It is necessary to maintain the reduction while a cast or splint is applied. In order to maintain your reduction, hold the wrist in a flexed, ulnarly deviated, and pronated position. We recommend cupping the elbow with one hand and grasping the digits with the other hand while maintaining slight traction. This position allows your assistant space to role a short arm cast or place a single sugar-tong splint (Fig. 4-21).
- While your assistant rolls the cast, the wrist should be in mild flexion, ulnar deviation, and pronation. As the cast material hardens, place a three point mold. We prefer to place one hand dorsally over the distal fragment, with the other hand volarly just proximal to the fracture, and a knee dorsally over the proximal forearm (Fig. 4-22). (An alternative technique is described below in the tricks section.)

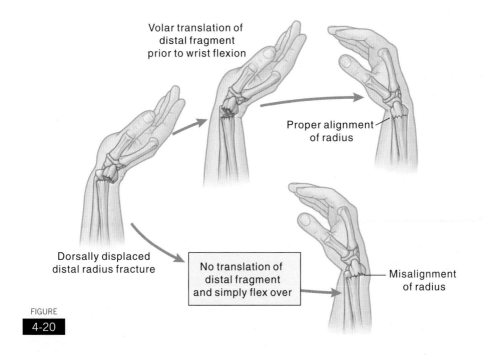

Volar translation of distal fragment prior to wrist flexion

Proper alignment of radius

Dorsally displaced distal radius fracture

No translation of distal fragment and simply flex over

Misalignment of radius

FIGURE
4-20

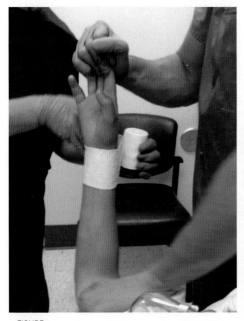

FIGURE
4-21

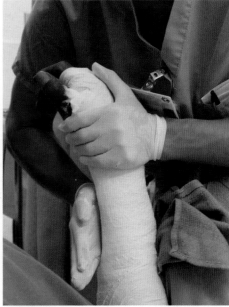

FIGURE
4-22

Fingertraps Technique

- Place the patient supine with the contralateral shoulder at the edge of the bed. Apply a strip of tape from the volar surface of the digit wrapping around the fingertip to the dorsum for easy trap removal.
- Place the hand in fingertraps. Only the thumb, index finger and middle finger are placed in traps to achieve ulnar deviation.
- Hang 10 to 15 lb of weight from the patients arm with the elbow at 90°. Wait 10 minutes to allow for muscular relaxation (Fig. 4-23).
- Usually, sufficient radial height will be obtained after 10 minutes; therefore, dorsal displacement can be corrected by using both thumbs on the dorsum of the radius to push the fragment volarly. A single sugar-tong splint or short arm cast can be applied prior to release of traction (Fig. 4-24).
- If radial height is not acceptable, then a brief period of increased traction can be applied. Typically, we leave the hand in traps and the weight applied while manually pushing the arm toward the floor.

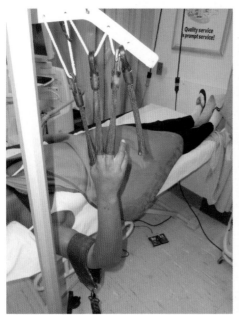

FIGURE
4-23

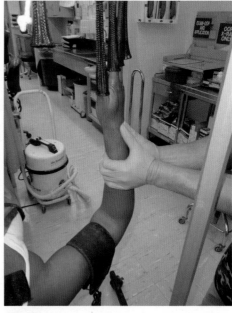

FIGURE
4-24

Sheet Technique

- The patient lies supine with the elbow at 90°. A sheet is draped around the arm so the free ends of the sheet are near the floor. Use your foot to step on the sheets pinning them to the floor. Now you can pull traction against the sheet (Fig. 4-25).

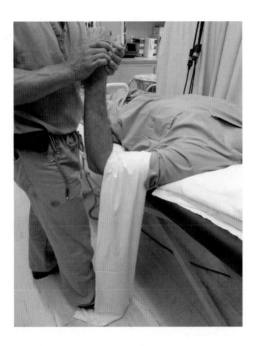

FIGURE
4-25

Tips and Other Considerations

▪ Be cautious in patients with fragile dorsal skin (e.g., elderly patients) since aggressive reduction maneuvers are likely to result in skin tears. In these patients, use less force, and attempt to minimize shear forces across the skin.

▪ When placing the 3-point mold focus on translating the distal fragment, rather than flexing the wrist. This maneuver takes practice but is critical in the nonoperative treatment of distal radius fractures.

▪ Do not immobilize patients in excessive wrist flexion, pronation, and ulnar deviation. While you may be more successful in maintaining the reduction, it is likely for the patient to develop digital stiffness, chronic region pain syndrome, and/or median nerve injury.

Perilunate Dislocation

Indication

Nearly (see other considerations) all perilunate dislocations require urgent closed reduction to reduce median nerve compression. However, surgical treatment is usually chosen for definitive treatment. The key to reduction of perilunate dislocations is understanding that in the early stages the carpal bones dislocate dorsally around a normally positioned lunate. In the final stage, the lunate is pushed volarly into the carpal tunnel, and the head of the capitate rests within the lunate fossa of the distal radius.

Description of Procedure

▪ A large amount of traction is occasionally required, therefore we often combine conscious sedation with an intra-articular wrist injection of 3 cc 1% lidocaine without epinephrine. In patients that present immediately after injury, a hematoma aspiration and intra-articular wrist injection may be sufficient.

- Position the patient supine with the shoulder at the edge of the bed and the elbow flexed. Perform the intra-articular wrist block. Place the patient in finger traps and apply 15 lb of traction for 15 minutes (as described in distal radius section).
- *Optional*: Administer conscious sedation if manipulation of the patient's wrist is uncomfortable.
- The approach to closed reduction changes depending on the position of the lunate.
  - If the lunate is positioned in its anatomic position, the wrist is hyperextended with concomitant application of traction. Specifically use one hand to pull traction while placing the thumb of your other hand on the head of the capitate. The lunate must be held in a reduced position with volar pressure. Now pull firm traction and push the head of the capitate dorsally as the wrist is flexed. The wrist will reduce with a palpable clunk (Figs. 4-26 and 4-27).
  - If the lunate is initially dislocated, start in a similar manner by placing the patient in fingertraps. However, the goal is to reduce the lunate first. For these maneuvers we leave the patient in fingertraps. Flex the wrist, and place your thumb on the volarly dislocated lunate. It is easiest to locate the lunate by placing your thumb just distal to the distal transverse wrist crease. With the wrist flexed, push the lunate dorsally and distally. Now proceed with reduction of the head of the capitate using the finger traps to maintain traction while you hyperextend the wrist. Be sure to keep your thumb volarly on the lunate to prevent inadvertent redislocation of the lunate by the head of

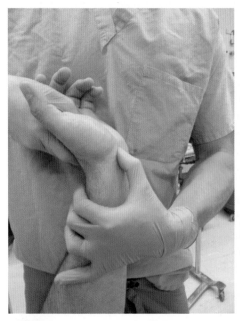

FIGURE

4-26

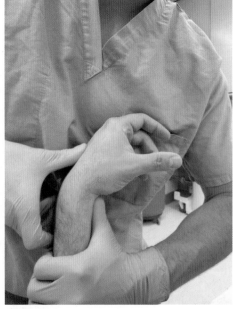

FIGURE

4-27

the capitate. As the wrist is brought from hyperextension to flexion, the reduction is often felt as a palpable clunk.

■ Because this is a hyperextension injury, the wrist is immobilized in flexion. To avoid median nerve dysfunction we always immobilize the wrist in <30° of flexion. Depending on the amount of swelling present, a single sugar-tong splint or a short arm cast can be used.

Tips and Other Considerations

■ When the lunate is volarly dislocated, there are three ways to ensure that the head of the capitate does not rotate the lunate out of the lunate fossa. First, adequate traction is required. Next and most importantly, maximal hyperextension should be obtained during the reduction maneuver. Finally, a thumb volarly on the lunate may prevent rotation.

■ Some surgeons discourage closed reduction attempts when the lunate is rotated >90° out of the fossa (the spilled teacup sign) because there is a theoretical risk of additional ligamentous and vascular injury. Approach these cases with caution. If the patient has median nerve symptoms, it may still be desirable to perform a closed reduction, but it must be done gently.

Metacarpal Fractures

Indication

Closed reduction is indicated for fractures of the index or middle finger metacarpals that are angulated >10° and ring or small finger fractures that are angulated >30° to 40°. Fractures of the metacarpal shaft have slightly more stringent indications. Additionally, any rotation deformity should be identified and corrected.

Tolerances

■ Index and middle fingers: <40° to 70° (neck), <30° (shaft).
■ Ring and small fingers: <10° (neck), <5° (shaft).

Description of Procedure

■ A hematoma block is utilized for anesthesia during reduction of metacarpal fractures. Usually there is a palpable step-off, which allows for easy needle placement. A 22G or 25G needle is advanced into the fracture site and 2 to 3 mL of 1% lidocaine is injected.

■ *Optional*: First attempt the reduction under fluoroscopy. Important information gleaned from fluoroscopy is the position of the dorsal mold and the optimal amount of MCP joint flexion.

■ At this point, the provisional reduction is ignored. A short arm cast is applied with the wrist in 15° of extension. Make sure that the dorsal portion of the plaster is sufficiently distal to allow for a dorsal mode yet low enough volarly to allow for proper placement of the outrigger. The cast is wrapped obliquely high dorsal to low volar.

■ Place the outrigger distally enough that it supports the finger but low enough that it allows 90° of flexion. Typically, the outrigger sits just below the level of the distal transverse wrist crease. If it is distal to this crease, the digit is pulled over the outrigger accentuating the deformity (Fig. 4-28).

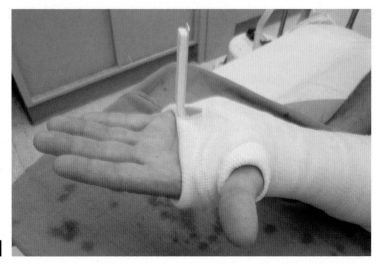

FIGURE

4-28

- Next, mold the cast using the palm of your hand on the dorsum just distal to the apex of the fracture and thumb pressure on the volarly placed outrigger (Fig. 4-29).
- Finally, perform your definitive reduction. Flex the MCP joint to the predetermined degree (usually 90°) with the interphalangeal joints fully straight. Use the base of the proximal phalanx as a battering ram to correct the flexion deformity of the metacarpal neck or shaft (Fig. 4-30).
- Match the rotation of the injured finger to that of the uninjured hand by rotating the digit in the same position.
- Tape the finger securely to the outrigger in the reduced position (Fig. 4-31).

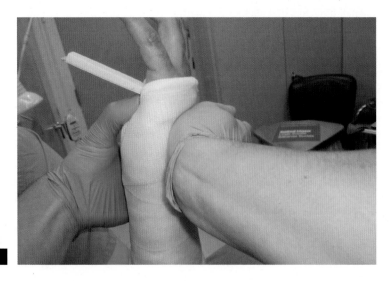

FIGURE

4-29

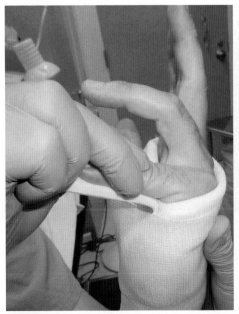

FIGURE
4-30

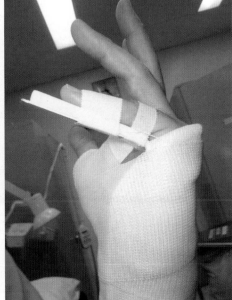

FIGURE
4-31

Tips

- In some metacarpal shaft fractures, as opposed to metacarpal neck fractures, the reduction is more easily obtained at 45° to 70° of MCP joint flexion. Fluoroscopy is useful to determine the optimal position in these cases.
- Either an ulnar gutter splint or short arm cast with an outrigger can be used to maintain the reduction. While placing the cast, make sure that the MCP joint is properly flexed and the interphalangeal joints are fully extended.
- For fractures at the base of the metacarpal and dislocations of the carpometacarpal (CMC) joint, an outrigger may not be necessary. In these cases, a short arm cast with a well-performed mold is usually sufficient. However, for these injuries extension of the wrist is particularly important.
- Although the temptation is great, especially in difficult fractures, never use your thumb to place the dorsal mold. We have seen disastrous skin complications as a result of aggressive digital pressure during cast molding for metacarpal fractures. However, we have not had any complications when gentle thumb pressure is placed volarly over a properly placed outrigger.
- You must match the rotation of the fractured metacarpal to that of the other hand. Most commonly, all digits point to the distal pole of the scaphoid, however individual variation exists. Therefore, prior to performing a reduction examine the uninjured hand as a guide to proper rotation. To assess rotation of the uninjured finger have the patient slowly flex their fingers as you observe the rotational alignment. Malrotation deformity can result in disabling scissoring of the fingers with grip (Fig. 4-32).

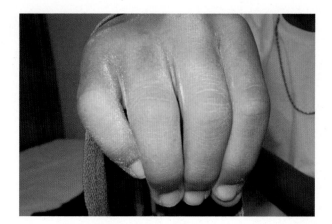

FIGURE
4-32

Bennett Fractures

Indications

The Bennett fracture is a fracture dislocation of the first CMC joint. A variably sized portion of the volar ulnar base of the first metacarpal remains attached to the trapezium via the volar oblique ligament. The remainder of the base of the first metacarpal subluxates dorsoradially and proximally. Although most Bennett fractures are unstable, closed reduction and immobilization can be used as definitive treatment in select cases. The primary deforming forces are the abductor pollicis longus and adductor pollicis, which result in supination, shortening, and dorsoradial displacement.

Description of Procedure

- For anesthesia, we prefer an injection of 1% lidocaine into the first CMC joint. Because the joint is subluxated, it is often difficult to use surface landmarks to accurately place the needle. For this reason, fluoroscopy is helpful to guide the needle into the joint.
- For traction, either apply a single finger trap to the thumb or pull manual traction.
- The first step of the reduction is to appose the fracture surfaces. To achieve this, position the thumb in pronation and abduction, while pulling traction as above (Fig. 4-33).

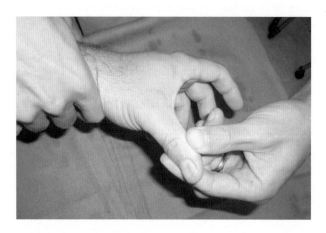

FIGURE
4-33

- Place the thumb of your other hand on the dorsoradial aspect of the thumb metacarpal, and reduce the joint subluxation by pushing the base of the thumb volarly and ulnarly. While an adequate reduction maybe palpable, we use fluoroscopy to confirm reduction (Fig. 4-34).
- Place a short-arm thumb spica cast while holding the thumb in the reduced position. A dorsoradial mold is placed with the palm of your hand to resist redisplacement (Fig. 4-35).

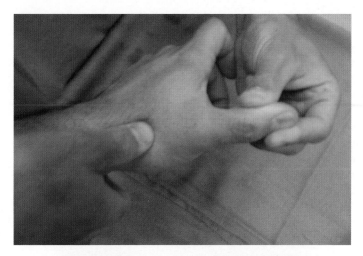

FIGURE
4-34

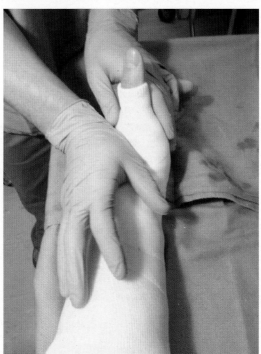

FIGURE
4-35

Phalangeal Fractures

Indications

This section will focus on extraarticular proximal phalanx fractures; however, discussion of middle and distal phalanx fractures can be found in the "other considerations" section. The closed treatment of proximal phalanx fractures is guided by two principles. Stability is primarily determined by bony length stability since an acceptable reduction can be obtained and maintained in most length stable fractures. Second, it is important to understand the primary deforming forces. Invariably, an apex volar deformity is present. The interossei muscles insert on the base of the proximal phalanx pulling the proximal fragment into flexion, while the central slip inserts on the base of the middle phalanx pulling the distal fragment into extension. The combination of these forces results in the extension or apex volar angulation.

Tolerances (extraarticular proximal phalanx fractures)

- angulation <10°
- shortening <2 mm
- translation <50%
- no malrotation

Description of Procedure

- We perform these reductions under a digital nerve block. The flexor tendon sheath block is our preferred method; however, supplementation with a dorsal digital block is occasionally required.
- The first step of treatment is to restore the length of the proximal phalanx. This step can be achieved by manual traction or a single finger trap (Fig. 4-36).
- Once the proximal phalanx is out to length, the most critical portion of the procedure is to flex the MCP joint to 90° while keeping both IP joints straight. This relaxes the deforming forces of the intrinsic muscles and is oftentimes all you need to complete the reduction (Fig. 4-37).

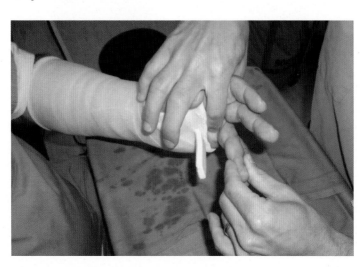

FIGURE
4-36

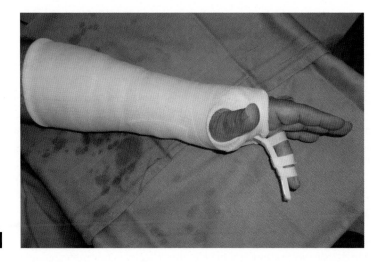

FIGURE
4-37

- Also note the rotation of the digit and ensure that it is equal to the contralateral unin-jured finger. Correction of malrotation is easily performed with the digit in this position.
- It is important to recognize that to properly stabilize these fractures you must immobilize the MCP joint as well as interphalangeal (IP) joints. Our preference is to use a short arm cast with an outrigger. Other alternatives include an ulnar gutter splint for the ring and small finger or a radial gutter splint for the middle and index fingers.

Tips and Other Considerations

- Occasionally, radial or ulnar angulation is difficult to correct. This issue is most fre-quently seen in base of the proximal phalanx fractures. To achieve coronal plane reduc-tion, it can be useful to place a pencil in the webspace to use as a fulcrum.
- The technique described above is best used for stable fractures that involve the shaft of the proximal phalanx. Intra-articular fractures, either unicondylar or bicondylar, tend to be highly unstable and usually require operative treatment. While nondisplaced unicon-dylar fractures can be treated nonoperatively, they require close follow-up and a compli-ant patient to prevent late displacement.
- Middle phalanx fractures have more variable angulation, depending on the location of the fracture relative to the flexor digitorum superficialis and central slip insertions. Nonetheless, the reduction technique is the same as proximal phalanx fractures.
- Distal phalanx fractures typically fall into two varieties. These are both described in the following sections on mallet fingers and fingertip injuries.

Digital Dislocations

Indications

All acute digital dislocations should be reduced. The MCP, proximal interphalangeal (PIP) and distal interphalangeal (DIP) joints are most commonly dislocated dorsally due to a hy-perextension injury. When approaching a closed reduction of any of the joints in the finger, it is important to perform reduction maneuvers in such a way that you do not convert a simple dislocation into an irreducible dislocation, which requires surgical treatment.

Description of Procedure: Proximal Interphalangeal Joint Dorsal Dislocation

- A digital nerve block is performed for anesthesia during the procedure.
- Grasp the finger distal to the PIP joint and apply only enough traction so that the base of the middle phalanx clears the head of the proximal phalanx. Additional traction rarely helps with the reduction and risks opening a space to allow volar plate interposition, which will convert a simple dislocation into an irreducible dislocation (Figs. 4-38 and 4-39).
- Place your other thumb dorsally on the base of the middle phalanx. Push the middle phalanx distally and volarly over the head of the proximal phalanx as the PIP joint is brought into more flexion. The reduction will be obtained with a palpable clunk (Fig. 4-40).
- After the reduction is completed, perform a stability examine with attention to the degree of extension at which subluxation occurs. While stability testing can be performed using palpation to detect subluxation, if available, fluoroscopy is our preferred method.
- If the finger is absolutely stable, then you can simply buddy tape to the adjacent digit, and start early range of motion. If any instability in extension is demonstrated, then place a dorsal blocking splint. We apply this splint only immobilizing the PIP joint (leaving the DIP and MCP joints free) with a 20° flexion safety stop (if the PIP joint subluxates at 10° of flexion, then we splint with a block at 30° of flexion) (Fig. 4-41).

Tips and Other Considerations

- In the case of a volarly dislocated PIP joint, rupture of the central slip portion of the extensor mechanism is common. In these cases, a hand surgery consult should be obtained.
- To reduce dorsal DIP joint dislocations, follow the same steps as for a PIP joint dislocation.

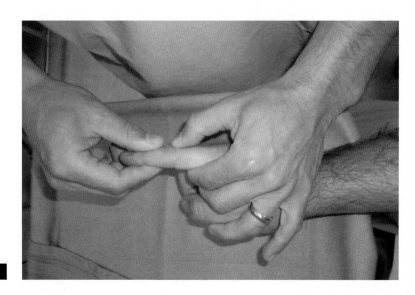

FIGURE
4-38

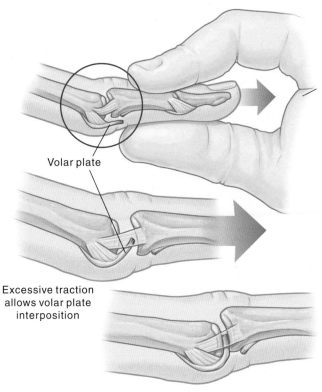

Volar plate

Excessive traction
allows volar plate
interposition

Irreducible dislocation

FIGURE
4-39

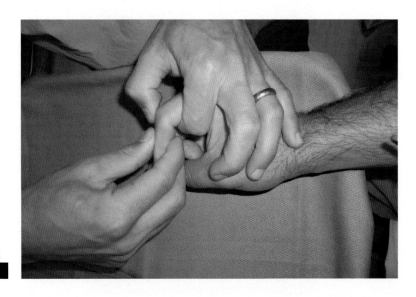

FIGURE
4-40

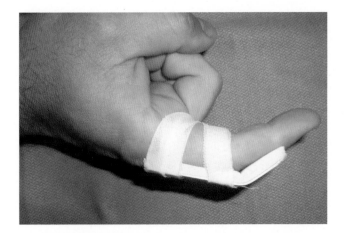

FIGURE

4-41

Description of Procedure: Metacarpophalangeal Joint Dorsal Dislocation

In dorsal MCP joint dislocations, there are two possible soft tissue impediments to reduction. The first is the invariably torn volar plate. The second are the flexor tendons and intrinsic muscles, which can act as noose around the metacarpal head.

- Typically, either a proximally placed digital nerve block or an intraarticular injection can be used for anesthesia during reductions of the MCP joint.
- It is critical to flex both the wrist and IP joints to relax the flexor tendons during reduction. This makes it less likely for the flexor tendons to form a noose around the metacarpal head. With the hand in this position, hyperextend only the MCP joint (Fig. 4-42).

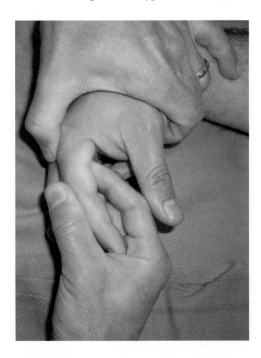

FIGURE

4-42

With very little traction, use your thumb to push the base of the proximal phalanx over and around the metacarpal head.

- Similar to the PIP joint dislocation, test joint stability clinically or with fluoroscopy to determine method of immobilization.
- Most commonly, the MCP joint is stable after reduction, and simple buddy taping will suffice. In cases where extension instability exists, use a dorsal blocking splint to prevent hyperextension.

Tips and Other Considerations

- Volar plate interposition is common in MCP joint dislocations, therefore minimal traction should be applied. Most of the reduction is done with the dorsally placed thumb. As your thumb slides the base of proximal phalanx over articular surface, it also pushes the volar plate away from the joint. Excessive traction will actually open the joint space, allowing for the volar plate to become interposed.

Mallet Finger

Indication

A mallet finger is a disruption of the terminal extensor tendon to the digit. The patient will be unable to extend the DIP joint secondary to a pure soft tissue disruption of the tendon or a variably sized avulsion fracture. Most acute and chronic mallet fingers are initially treated nonoperatively.

Description of Procedure

- Mallet fingers are treated in extension for 6 to 8 weeks. We prefer to treat this injury in slight hyperextension.
- Examine the contralateral digit to determine the amount of passive hyperextension of the DIP joint that exists in your particular patient. The injured finger will be splinted in less than 50% of the contralateral maximal hyperextension. For instance, if the patient can passively hyperextend 30°, then splint the injured digit in 15° of hyperextension or less.
- A number of splints can be used to maintain the DIP joint in hyperextension. The splint should only immobilize the DIP joint leaving the other joints free. Specific splints include the stack splint, thermoplastic splint, and aluminum foam splint.
- Our preference is to mold an aluminum foam splint to achieve the desired amount of hyperextension based on individual patient. The splint is best placed volarly and secured with cloth tape (Fig. 4-43).
- The DIP joint is splinted in extension 24 hours per day for 8 weeks. Then the patient uses a night splint for an additional 2 to 4 weeks.

Tips and Other Considerations

- Do not force the digit into maximal hyperextension because it can cause vascular compromise and dorsal skin breakdown.
- The patient should be instructed on how to remove the splint and clean the digit without letting the DIP joint flex. If inadvertent flexion occurs, then the course of immobilization restarts.

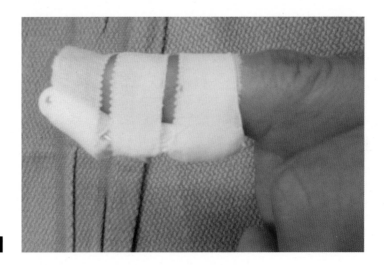

FIGURE
4-43

- These patients should follow-up in less than 1 week to ensure compliance with immobilization and to check for vascular or skin problems.
- Occasionally, a large bony avulsion fragment is present. This is only an indication for surgery if the joint subluxates in extension. Therefore, in these cases, a radiograph should be obtained after splint placement. If only mild subluxation occurs, then the amount of hyperextension can be reduced, but the finger should never be splinted in any flexion.

PROCEDURES

Fingertip Injuries

Indication

Fingertip injuries can involve a number of different anatomic structures including the distal phalanx, nail bed, and skin/subcutaneous tissue. When approaching these injuries, first determine if there is sufficient amount of skin to cover the bone of the distal phalanx.

Description of Procedure

- Perform a digital nerve block for anesthesia during the procedure.
- Perform an initial irrigation of the wound. This can be done with sterile saline; however, the patient can simply hold the fingertip under a running faucet for 5 minutes.
- Sterilely prep and drape the hand with a Betadine solution. Use a penrose drain or elastic tourniquet for a blood-free field. We always use a clamp to secure the tourniquet because it makes it less likely to forget to remove it at the end of the procedure.
- Assess the wound and debride any devitalized tissue. Determine if the nail bed is injured and whether adequate soft tissue exists for a tension free closure.
- Patients usually fit in one of three categories:
  - Patient 1: If a sufficient amount of the nail bed remains and the soft tissue cannot be closed over the distal phalanx, then the patient will need operative treatment for soft

tissue coverage. This is the patient that requires full length of the digit, but does not have sufficient soft tissue coverage. We do not recommend performing skin grafts or local flaps in the emergency room.

- Patient 2: A nail bed injury is present and no bone is exposed. In this patient, perform a nail bed repair (described below). The skin can be closed with suture (described below) or left open and allowed to heal by secondary intention. In general, if the wound is <1 cm^2, we let it heal by secondary intention. If the wound is >1 cm^2, then it should be closed with suture.
- Patient 3: The nail bed is insufficient to produce a nail and bone is exposed. In this case, length is not important because a distal phalanx is not needed to support the nail bed. In these cases, we remove enough bone of the distal phalanx to allow for a primary closure (described below).

- Removal of exposed distal phalanx:
  - If indicated, you can remove a variable amount of bone with the use of a rongeur or bone cutter. Both instruments are stocked in most operating rooms.
  - If a rongeur is chosen, then nibble down the jagged ends of the cortical rim of the distal phalanx to the desired level. When using the rongeur, make sure to squeeze the handle hard so that accurate bone resection is achieved. Do not rely on leverage to snap off bone fragments, since this technique is less accurate.
  - If a bone cutter is chosen, then grasp the entire distal phalanx at the desired level and make a transverse flat resection. Ensure that the cutter is sharp because a dull instrument will crush the distal phalanx rather than transecting it. If needed, use the cutter to smooth the bony edges.

- Nail bed repair:
  - To perform a nail bed repair, the nail must first be removed. We use a freer elevator to atraumatically separate the nail from its bed. The nail is placed in a saline bath, so it can be used later in the procedure. If a freer elevator is not available, then iris scissors can be used to separate the nail and are available in most emergency rooms.
  - Use fine absorbable monofilament suture to repair the nail bed. Or preference is 6-0 plain gut, however other alternatives exist.
  - Simple interrupted sutures are preferred. We do not use loupe magnification for the repair. Only three throws are made for the knot and the ends are cut close to the knot. A low profile knot makes it easier to replace the nail over your repair.
  - In cases where the nail is not badly damaged, remove it from the saline bath and replace it underneath of the nail fold. It must be secured at the periphery with five simple interrupted sutures using 4-0 nylon on a cutting needle. Two sutures are placed on each side of the nail and one at the tip of the nail. The sutures are first placed through the nail (reason that a cutting needle is required) and then through the skin on the adjacent to the nail bed. Replacing the nail serves two purposes: protection of the nail bed repair, and ensuring that the nail fold does not prematurely close which can prevent nail formation.
  - If the nail is badly damaged, then we cut out a nail-shaped piece of aluminum foil (certain packaging materials from dressing supplies can be used), and this is used in place of a nail.

- Skin coverage:
  - We do not advocate performing any local flaps or skin grafts in the emergency room.
  - All skin closure is performed in the emergency room in a tension-free manner with 4-0 or 5-0 absorbable sutures. Simple interrupted sutures are preferred.
  - Some studies suggest that healing by secondary intention may have better results. If you intend to allow the wound to heal by secondary intention, then either wet to dry dressing changes can be used, or a petroleum impregnated dressing can be placed over the defect.

Tips and Other Considerations

- The described procedures are only for injuries distal to the DIP joint. For injuries at or proximal to the DIP joint, a hand surgery consult should be obtained to evaluate the patient for reimplantation.

Compartment Pressure Measurement in the Hand

Indication

Compartment syndrome occurs when the pressure within the fascial compartment exceeds capillary pressure, leading to tissue ischemia. It is an orthopaedic emergency and requires emergent fasciotomy. The use of compartment pressure measurement in the diagnosis of compartment syndrome is controversial. Because false negatives and false positives can occur, pressure measurements can fluctuate with time and proximity to the traumatized tissue, and the pressure that defines compartment syndrome is unknown, we prefer to make the diagnosis on the basis of clinical examination when possible. Compartment pressure measurement is utilized when the patient is intoxicated, obtunded, or otherwise incapable with cooperating with an examination. When performed, we define compartment syndrome when the compartment pressure is within 30 mm Hg of the patient's diastolic blood pressure.

Description of Procedure

- The hand contains 11 compartments: 7 interossei (3 volar, 4 dorsal), hypothenar, thenar, adductor, and carpal tunnel (Fig. 4-44).
- Position the patient supine.
- Prepare a wide area of the skin with antibacterial solution.
- *Optional:* Mark the entry site with a marking pen. Perform this step prior to application of antibacterial solution if a nonsterile pen is used.
- Three entry sites are required to access the compartments of the hand.
  - Dorsal interossei: The entry site is located on the dorsum of the hand 1cm proximal to the metacarpal head. The needle is inserted 1 to 2 cm until the muscle belly of the dorsal interossei is felt. The actual insertion depth varies depending on the amount of dorsal soft tissue swelling (Fig. 4-45).
  - Volar interossei: Using the same insertion, simply advance the needle 0.5 to 1 cm more volar to assess the volar interossei muscle.
  - Adductor: Insert the needle 2 cm distal to the index finger metacarpal head. The insertion site is on the radial side of the index finger metacarpal in the first webspace (Fig. 4-46).

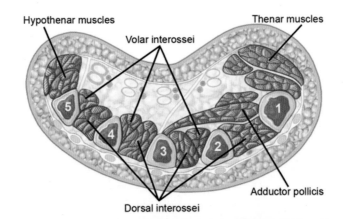

FIGURE
4-44

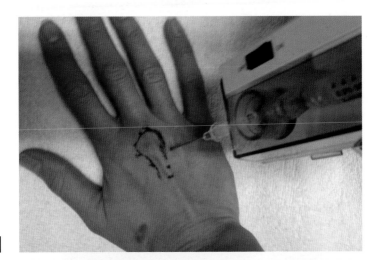

FIGURE
4-45

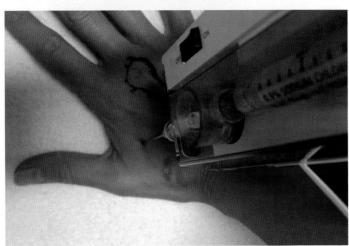

FIGURE
4-46

■ Hypothenar and thenar: Insert the needle at the respective glabrous–nonglabrous skin junction of the ulnar and radial sides of the hand. The needle is inserted 1cm into the muscular eminence (Figs. 4-47 and 4-48).

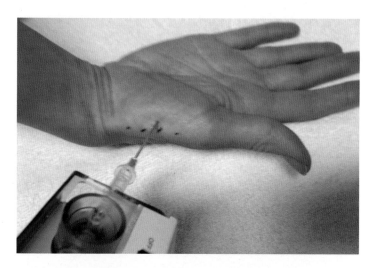

FIGURE
4-47

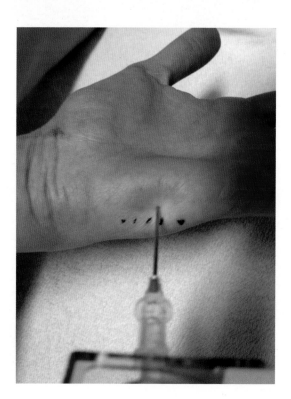

FIGURE
4-48

▓ *Optional:* Anesthetize the skin overlying the planned entry site with 2 to 3 mL of local anesthetic.

▓ Assemble the intracompartmental pressure measuring device according to the manufacturer's specifications (Fig. 4-49). Alternatively, an arterial line system with high pressure tubing and a wick or slit catheter can be used (Fig. 4-50).

▓ Hold the needle/pressure transducer at the level of the entry site and at the angle of insertion. Zero the system.

Tips and Other Considerations

To determine the proper insertion depth, use a sterile marking pen to place 0.5, 1, and 1.5 cm hash marks on the needle.

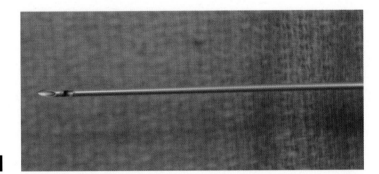

FIGURE
4-49

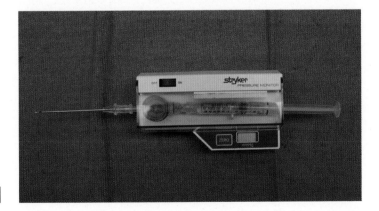

FIGURE
4-50

FIGURE CREDITS

Figure 4-44   From Wiesel SW. *Wiesel Operative Techniques in Orthopaedic Surgery.* Philadelphia, PA: Lippincott Williams & Wilkins; 2010.

5

The Pelvis, Hip, and Thigh

INJECTIONS AND ASPIRATIONS

Intra-articular Hip Injection/Aspiration

Indication

Intra-articular positioning of a needle is useful for aspirating fluid for laboratory analysis, injecting arthrogram dye, and medication delivery. In adults, a lateral or anterolateral approach is commonly used; in children, the medial approach is preferred.

Description of Procedure

LATERAL APPROACH

- Position the patient supine on a bed or gurney.
- Prepare a wide area of the skin at the lateral aspect of the hip with antibacterial solution.
- *Optional:* Mark the entry site with a marking pen. Perform this step before application of antibacterial solution if a nonsterile pen is used.
- The entry site is 2 cm distal to the tip of the greater trochanter on its palpable anterior border (Fig. 5-1).
- *Optional:* Anesthetize the skin overlying the planned entry site with 2 to 3 mL of local anesthetic.
- Direct the needle parallel to the floor and perpendicular to the femur until bone is felt. The needle is now at the base of the femoral neck.
- Pull the needle back a few millimeters, and redirect at an angle directed approximately 10° anteriorly to match femoral anteversion and 45° superiorly to match the neck–shaft angle (Figs. 5-2 and Fig. 5-3).
- Advance the needle until bone is felt.
- Withdraw synovial fluid to verify intra-articular position of the needle.
- Continue aspirating or inject the desired fluid.

ANTEROLATERAL APPROACH

- Position the patient supine on a bed or gurney.
- Prepare a wide area of the skin at the anterolateral aspect of the hip with antibacterial solution.
- *Optional:* Mark the entry site with a marking pen. Perform this step before application of antibacterial solution if a nonsterile pen is used.

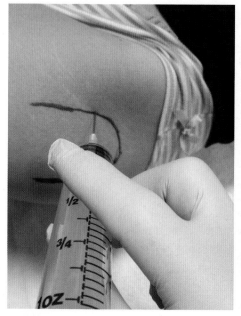

FIGURE
5-1

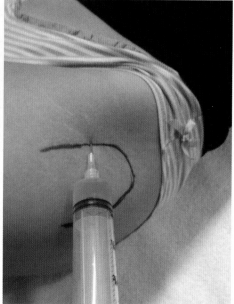

FIGURE
5-2

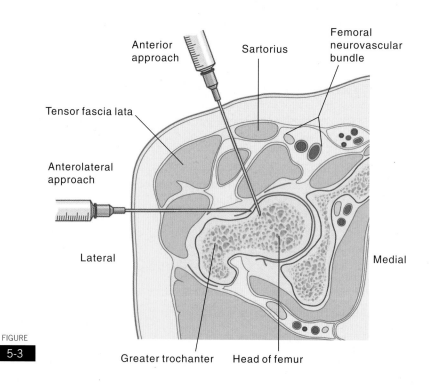

FIGURE
5-3

- Before needle insertion, palpate and mark the femoral artery pulse and ensure that you enter lateral to this structure and the adjacent femoral nerve.
- The entry site is located two fingerbreadths directly distal to the palpable anterior superior iliac spine (ASIS). If the needle is inserted perpendicular to the skin from this point, it will pierce the hip capsule at the femoral head/neck junction (Fig. 5-4).
- *Optional:* Anesthetize the skin overlying the planned entry site with 2 to 3 mL of local anesthetic.
- Direct the needle toward the femoral head/neck junction until bone is felt (Figs. 5-3 and 5-5).
- Pull the needle back a few millimeters and attempt aspiration.
- If no fluid is obtained, direct the needle inferiorly, just below the neck and advance more posterior. Since the patient is supine, the synovial fluid has a tendency to pool posteriorly, and it may be easier to obtain fluid in this location.
- Withdraw synovial fluid to verify intra-articular position of the needle.
- Continue aspirating or inject the desired fluid.

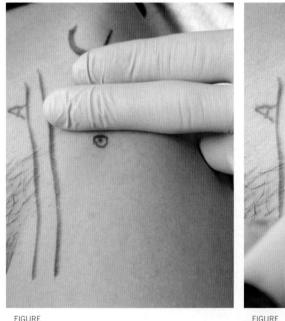

FIGURE
5-4

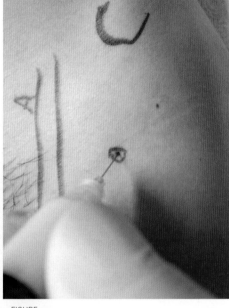

FIGURE
5-5

MEDIAL APPROACH

- Position the patient supine with the limb in the frog-leg position (abduction and external rotation).
- As this approach is typically utilized in a child, conscious sedation or general anesthesia is the preferred method of anesthesia.

- Prepare a wide area of the skin at the medial aspect of the hip with antibacterial solution.
- *Optional:* Mark the entry site with a marking pen. Perform this step before application of antibacterial solution if a nonsterile pen is used.
- The entry site is just deep to the easily palpable adductor longus tendon and 2 to 4 cm inferior to the pubic symphysis (based on the size of the child) (Figs. 5-6 and 5-7).
- Direct the needle parallel to the floor and toward the ASIS until bone is felt.
- Withdraw synovial fluid to verify intra-articular position of the needle.
- Continue aspirating or inject the desired fluid.

Tips and Other Considerations

- A rough estimate for the location of the center of the femoral head is a point two finger-breadths medial and one fingerbreadth inferior to the ASIS.
- A long spinal needle should always be used. The stylet should remain inside the needle whenever the needle is moved; otherwise, a core of tissue may obstruct the needle.
- When performing this procedure for the purposes of aspiration, an 18G needle is recommended, as inflammatory or septic fluid is quite viscous. For a corticosteroid solution injection, a smaller, 22G needle may be used, although the thinner needle is harder to direct.
- Because the hip joint is a deep structure, fluoroscopic guidance is often helpful in locating the hip. We prefer injection of radiopaque dye to confirm intra-articular placement before the administration of medications.

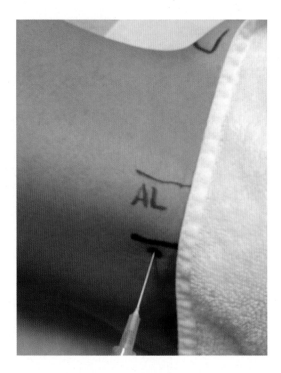

FIGURE

5-6

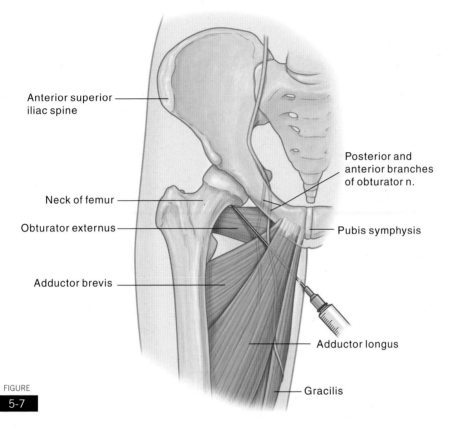

Anterior superior
iliac spine

Posterior and
anterior branches
of obturator n.

Neck of femur

Obturator externus

Pubis symphysis

Adductor brevis

Adductor longus

FIGURE
5-7

Gracilis

Trochanteric Bursa Injection/Aspiration

Indication

Placement of a needle within the trochanteric bursa permits aspiration of fluid for laboratory analysis or pain relief as well as the ability to inject local anesthetic and/or corticosteroid.

Description of Procedure

- Position the patient in the lateral decubitus position. Placement of the hip in slight abduction with a pillow or several towels between the legs will relax the iliotibial band.
- Prepare a wide area of the skin with antibacterial solution.
- *Optional:* Mark the entry site with a marking pen. Perform this step before application of antibacterial solution if a nonsterile pen is used.
- The entry site is over the palpable greater trochanter over the point of maximal tenderness (Fig. 5-8).
- *Optional:* Anesthetize the skin overlying the planned entry site with 2 to 3 mL of local anesthetic.
- Insert the needle to the point at which it contacts bone, and pull back slightly (1 to 2 mm).
- After aspirating to verify that the needle is not within a blood vessel, continue aspirating or inject the desired solution.

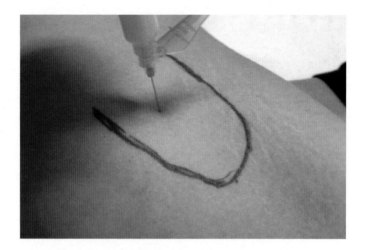

FIGURE
5-8

Tips and Other Considerations

- When performing this procedure for the purposes of aspiration, an 18G needle is recommended as inflammatory or septic fluid is quite viscous. For a corticosteroid solution injection, a smaller, 22G needle may be used.
- For many patients, a standard, 1.5-inch needle will be long enough to reach the trochanteric bursa; however, in larger individuals, a spinal needle is recommended.
- When injecting a corticosteroid/anesthetic solution for the treatment of trochanteric bursitis, greater pain relief may be achieved by injecting portions of the solution in slightly different positions because the bursa is septated and one injection site may not access the entire area.

CLOSED REDUCTIONS

Anterior–Posterior Compression Pelvic Fracture

Indication

The application of a pelvic binder or sheet can assist in the reduction of bony and venous hemorrhage, minimize pain, and provide provisional stabilization of pelvic fractures. Application of a pelvic binder or sheet is recommended in the setting of anterior–posterior compression (open book) pelvic fracture patterns. In a hemodynamically unstable patient with pelvic instability a pelvic binder or sheet should be placed as a life saving measure prior to radiographs. With lateral compression patterns, a theoretical risk of injury to intrapelvic structures (e.g. bladder, vaginal wall) exists; however, we feel that these risks are outweighed by the benefits of this potentially life saving intervention. In patients with a known (radiographs available) lateral compression injury, a binder is not recommended (Fig. 5-9).

Description of Procedure

- A minimum of two individuals are required for proper application.
- Center the binder or sheet under the patient at the level of the greater trochanters. Compression of the pelvic ring via the greater trochanters is more effective than the iliac crests (Fig. 5-10).

- While one or two providers apply an internal rotation force on the pelvis via the iliac crests, another provider secures the binder or sheet (Figs. 5-11 and 5-12).
- A sheet can be secured with several clamps or a knot.

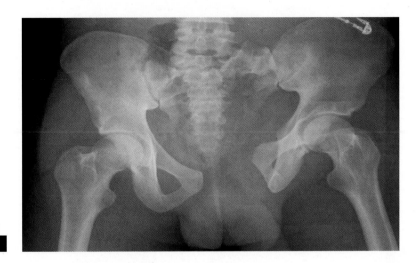

FIGURE
5-9

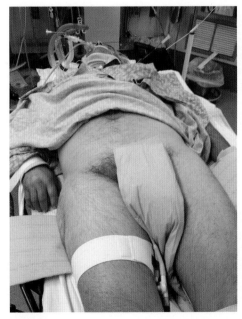

FIGURE
5-10

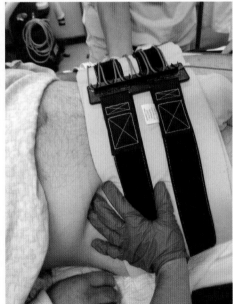

FIGURE
5-11

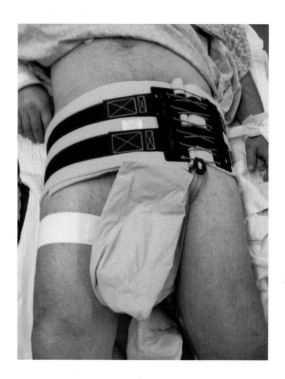

FIGURE
5-12

Tips and Other Considerations

- The most common error is to place the binder too superior, which is ineffective at maintaining pelvic ring reduction and causes compression of the abdomen resulting in difficulty with ventilation.
- Two options exist when the binder needs to be moved to access the groin or abdomen for angiography or exploratory laparotomy. A second binder can be placed around the mid to distal thigh, and the original pelvic binder can be removed. Alternatively, areas of the binder can be cut out to allow for sterile preparation without disrupting the integrity of the binder.
- When a sheet is used, avoid wrinkles, which can cause skin breakdown.

Hip Dislocation

Indication

The presence of an anterior (less common) or posterior dislocation of the femoral head, with or without the presence of associated acetabular or femoral head fractures, warrants an emergent attempt of closed reduction. The presence of a femoral neck fracture is a contraindication to closed reduction, as reduction attempts are both unlikely to be successful and likely to displace the fracture. While a dislocated hip arthroplasty still necessitates an urgent closed reduction, it is not considered a true emergency because the risk of osteonecrosis of the femoral head is not a concern.

Anterior Hip Dislocation

Description of Procedure

- Conscious sedation or general anesthesia is administered by the Emergency Department (ED) physician or anesthesiologist while the patient is supine on the bed or gurney.
- The general strategy is to use traction to get the femoral head over the lip of the acetabulum before rotating the hip back into the socket.
- Position the patient on the edge of the bed so that the leg can easily be abducted off the edge of the bed. Place a towel or sheet around the proximal thigh (Fig. 5-13).
- An assistant is required to stabilize the pelvis with direct pressure on bilateral ASISs.
- Apply traction in-line to the abducted and externally rotated limb. This brings the femoral head over the lip of the acetabulum (Fig. 5-14).

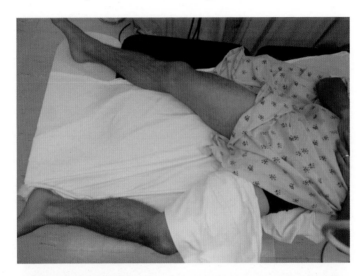

FIGURE
5-13

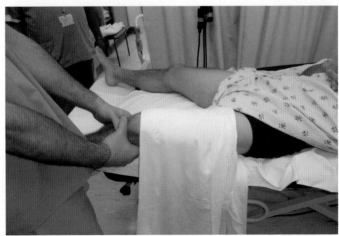

FIGURE
5-14

- Apply gentle internal rotation to direct the femoral head back into the acetabulum (Figs. 5-15 and 5-16).
- If reduction is still not achieved, laterally directed force to the thigh can be applied by an assistant with the towel around the thigh. Gentle, alternating internal and external rotation of the hip can also be attempted (Fig. 5-17).

Tips and Other Considerations

- Adequate relaxation is the most important component of this procedure. Choice of anesthetic is beyond the scope of this text; however, during the procedure it is important to guide the physician providing the sedation if resistance is felt.
- Always obtain adequate radiographs to rule out a femoral neck fracture before attempting a closed reduction.

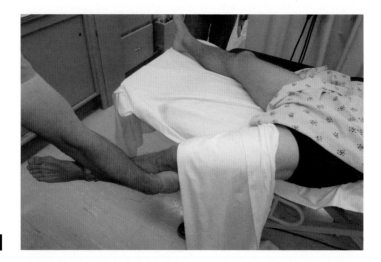

FIGURE

5-15

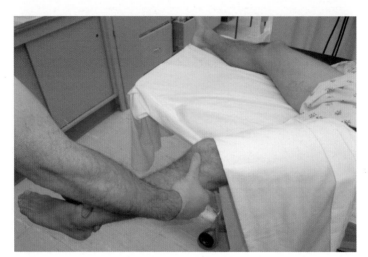

FIGURE

5-16

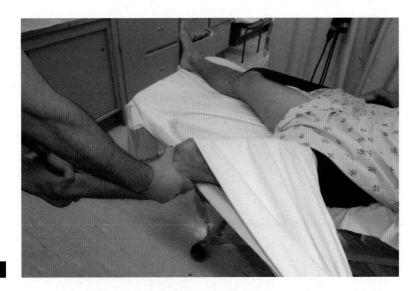

FIGURE
5-17

- Never forcibly rotate the hip. If the hip has not cleared the acetabular rim, then rotation of the hip can result in fracture of the proximal femur.
- Because the hip joint is relatively anterior with a minimal amount of overlying soft tissue, the femoral head is easily palpable in an anteriorly dislocated state. During the reduction maneuver while the hip is being internally rotated, have your assistant provide a posterior-laterally directed force to the femoral head to facilitate reduction.
- The reduction can be confirmed clinically by a freely mobile hip and equal leg lengths.
- After reduction, obtain an anteroposterior (AP) pelvis radiograph. If the reduction appears satisfactory on the radiograph, a CT of the hip is recommended to verify a concentric reduction and evaluate for intra-articular loose, bony fragments.

Posterior Hip Dislocation

Description of Procedure

ALLIS METHOD[1]

- Position the patient supine on a bed or gurney with a towel or sheet around the proximal thigh of the effected limb (Fig. 5-18).
- Conscious sedation or general anesthesia is administered by the ED physician or anesthesiologist.
- The physician should position himself standing on the patient's bed, straddling the lower extremities. An assistant is required to stabilize the pelvis with direct pressure on bilateral ASISs.
- Traction is applied in-line with the femur. Occasionally, reduction will be achieved with in-line traction alone (Fig. 5-19).
- While traction is maintained, slowly increase hip flexion to approximately 70° (Fig. 5-20).

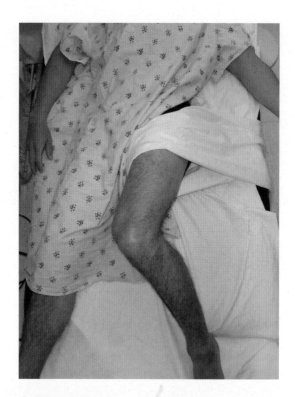

FIGURE
5-18

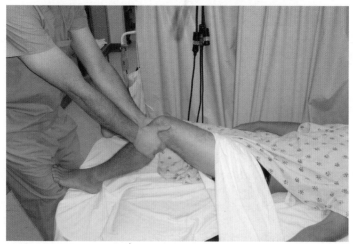

FIGURE
5-19

- Clearance over the posterior wall of the acetabulum can be facilitated with gentle internal and external rotation of the hip as well as having an assistant pull laterally on the towel around the thigh (Fig. 5-21).
- The reduction will be felt as a palpable clunk.
- After successful reduction, place an abduction pillow or several blankets or pillows between the patient's legs.

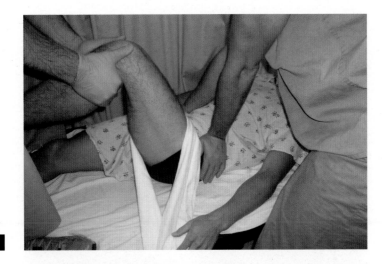

**FIGURE
5-20**

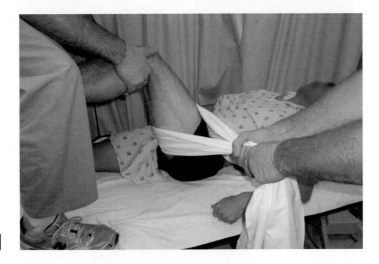

**FIGURE
5-21**

STIMSON GRAVITY METHOD[2]

- Conscious sedation or general anesthesia is administered by the ED physician or anesthesiologist while the patient is supine on the bed or gurney.
- Position the patient prone with the effected limb off the side of the bed or gurney. This position limits the use of this technique due to limited access to the airway.
- An assistant is required to stabilize the pelvis with direct pressure on bilateral posterior superior iliac spines (Fig. 5-22).
- Apply an anterior force on the posterior aspect of the proximal calf (Fig. 5-23).
- Clearance over the posterior wall of the acetabulum can be facilitated with gentle internal and external rotation of the hip (Fig. 5-24).
- After successful reduction, place an abduction pillow or several blankets or pillows between the patient's legs.

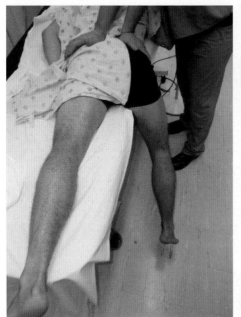

FIGURE
5-22

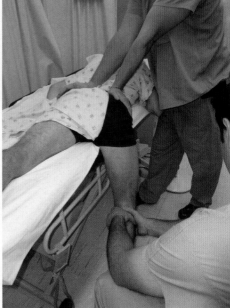

FIGURE
5-23

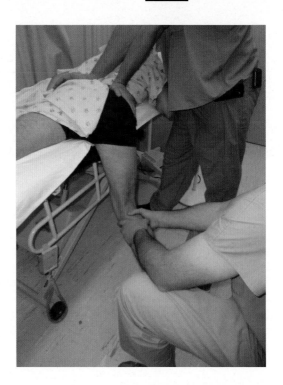

FIGURE
5-24

Tips and Other Considerations

- Adequate relaxation is the most important component of this procedure. Choice of anesthetic is beyond the scope of this text; however, during the procedure it is important to guide the physician providing the sedation if resistance is felt.
- Always obtain adequate radiographs to rule out a femoral neck fracture before attempting a closed reduction.
- Never forcibly rotate the hip. If the hip has not cleared the acetabular rim, then rotation of the hip can result in fracture of the proximal femur.
- The reduction can be confirmed clinically by a freely mobile hip and equal leg lengths.
- After you think that a reduction has been achieved, obtain an anteroposterior pelvis radiograph. If the reduction appears satisfactory on the radiograph, a CT of the hip is still recommended to verify a concentric reduction and evaluate for intra-articular loose, bony fragments.
- In the setting of intra-articular bony fragments or an unstable posterior wall fracture of the acetabulum, consider the application of skeletal traction (see "Distal Femoral Traction Pin").

PROCEDURES

Compartment Pressure Measurement in the Thigh

Indication

Compartment syndrome occurs when the pressure within the fascial compartment exceeds capillary pressure, leading to tissue ischemia. It is an orthopaedic emergency and requires emergent fasciotomy. The use of compartment pressure measurement in the diagnosis of compartment syndrome is controversial. Because false negatives and false positives can occur, pressure measurements can fluctuate with time and proximity to the traumatized tissue, and the pressure that defines compartment syndrome is unknown, we prefer to make the diagnosis on the basis of clinical examination when possible. Compartment pressure measurement is utilized when the patient is intoxicated, obtunded, or otherwise incapable of cooperating with an examination. When performed, we define compartment syndrome when the compartment pressure is within 30 mm Hg of the patient's diastolic blood pressure.

Description of Procedure

- The thigh contains three compartments: anterior, medial, and posterior (Fig. 5-25).
- Position the patient to allow access to the middle and proximal thigh.
- Prepare a wide area of the skin with antibacterial solution.
- *Optional:* Mark the entry site with a marking pen. Perform this step before application of antibacterial solution if a nonsterile pen is used.
- Each compartment requires a separate entry site.
  - Anterior Compartment: The entry site is located anterolateral over the prominent vastus lateralis in the mid thigh (Fig. 5-26).
  - Posterior Compartment: There are two ways to reach the posterior compartment. The same insertion site as the anterior compartment can be used. The needle is directed

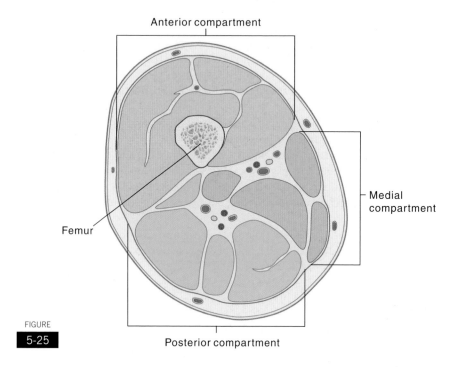

Anterior compartment

Medial compartment

Femur

Posterior compartment

FIGURE 5-25

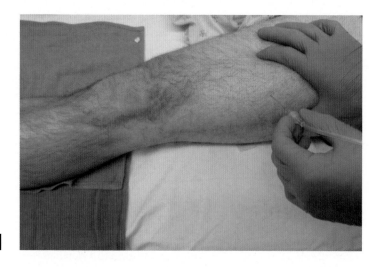

FIGURE 5-26

posteriorly until the intermuscular septum is pierced, indicating placement in the posterior compartment. Alternatively, a new insertion site two fingerbreadths posterior to the often palpable intermuscular septum can be used (Fig. 5-27).

■ Medial Compartment: The femoral artery is anterior at the level of the hip and branches with the superficial femoral artery coursing medially. Attempt to palpate this

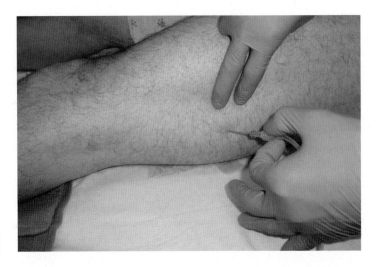

FIGURE
5-27

structure before insertion. Our preferred insertion site is the proximal medial thigh, which avoids the more lateral femoral neurovascular bundle. In the proximal third of the thigh, where the medial compartment musculature is the largest, the intermuscular septum between the anterior and medial compartments is often palpable. The entry site is approximately 1 to 2 cm medial/posterior to the intermuscular septum (Fig. 5-28).

- *Optional:* Anesthetize the skin overlying the planned entry site with 2 to 3 mL of local anesthetic.
- Assemble the intracompartmental pressure measuring device according to the manufacturer's specifications. Alternatively, an arterial line system with high-pressure tubing and a wick catheter can be used.
- Hold the needle/pressure transducer at the level of the entry site and at the angle of insertion. For each compartment, the angle will be such that the needle is directed centrally (toward the femur).

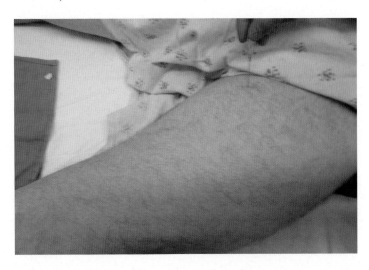

FIGURE
5-28

■ Zero the system.

■ Insert the needle approximately 2 to 3 cm.

■ Inject a very small (less than 1 mL) amount of fluid to clear tissue from the needle.

■ At this point, it is common for the pressure reading to become temporarily elevated before trending down and stabilizing at a value. Ensure enough passage of time to record a stable value, and avoid recording the initial, potentially falsely elevated value.

Tips and Other Considerations

■ For greatest accuracy, we recommend assessing the mean of three separate measurements in each compartment.

■ Proper positioning can be confirmed with the elevation of the pressure reading by the application of pressure over another portion of the compartment.

REFERENCES

1. Allis OH. XI. Everted Dorsal Dislocations of the Hip. *Ann Surg.* 1911;54(3):371–380.
2. Stimson LA. An Easy Method of Reducing Dislocations of the Shoulder and Hip. *New York Medical Record.* 1900;57(356).

6

The Knee and Leg

INJECTIONS AND ASPIRATIONS

Intra-articular Knee Injection/Aspiration

Indication

Intra-articular positioning of a needle allows the physician the ability to obtain synovial fluid for analysis, provide local anesthesia for procedures, evaluate for traumatic arthrotomy, and treat degenerative conditions with a variety of solutions.

Superomedial/Lateral Approach

Description of Procedure

- Position the patient supine with the knee in extension.
- Prepare a wide area of the skin with antibacterial solution.
- *Optional:* Mark the entry site with a marking pen. Perform this step before application of antibacterial solution if a nonsterile pen is used.
- The entry site is typically 1 cm medial or lateral to the respective border of the patella at the superior pole.
- *Optional:* Anesthetize the skin overlying the planned entry site with 2 to 3 mL of local anesthetic.
- Direct the needle through the skin into the suprapatellar pouch, which is between the patella and femur. If bony resistance is met, evaluate both your starting point and the angle of your needle and determine if you are encountering the patella or femur before making adjustments. The thickness of the patella is commonly underestimated (Figs. 6-1 and 6-2).

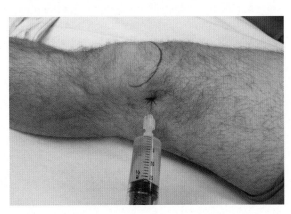

FIGURE
6-1

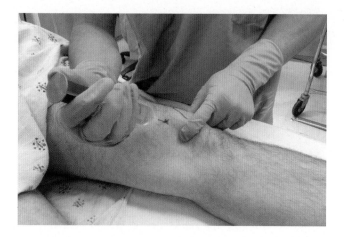

FIGURE
6-2

- Aspirate synovial fluid to verify that the needle is appropriately positioned.
- Continue aspirating or inject the desired solution.

Anteromedial/Lateral Approach

Description of Procedure

- Position the knee in 90° of flexion.
- Prepare a wide area of the skin with antibacterial solution.
- Palpate medial/lateral joint line and the medial/lateral boarder of the patellar tendon.
- *Optional:* Mark the entry site with a marking pen. Perform this step before application of antibacterial solution if a nonsterile pen is used.
- The entry site is approximately 1.5 cm proximal to the tibial plateau, just medial or lateral to the respective side of the patellar tendon. The joint line is typically palpable; however, the distal pole of the patella is a good landmark for the level of the joint (Fig. 6-3).
- *Optional:* Anesthetize the skin overlying the entry site with 2 to 3 mL of local anesthetic.
- Direct the needle through the skin into the anterolateral/medial area of the knee joint. If bony resistance is met, evaluate your position, withdraw the needle to the skin, and redirect. An entry site or angle too distal will cause you to hit the tibia, and an entry site or angle too proximal will cause you to hit the respective femoral condyle (Figs. 6-4 and 6-5).
- Aspirate synovial fluid to verify that the needle is appropriately positioned.
- Continue aspirating or inject the desired solution.

Tips and Other Considerations

- The use of local anesthetic is debatable. Some physicians feel it is not helpful because only the skin will be anesthetized and a second injection is required.
- For aspirations, an 18G needle with a large (35 mL or larger) syringe is generally recommended. For injections, a 22G needle with a smaller syringe may be used.
- Although advantages and disadvantages of the approaches can be debated, we typically perform injections via the anterolateral approach and aspirations via the superolateral approach.

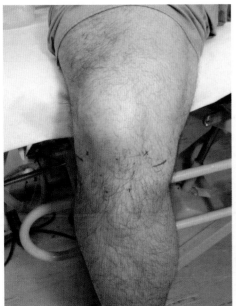

FIGURE
6-3

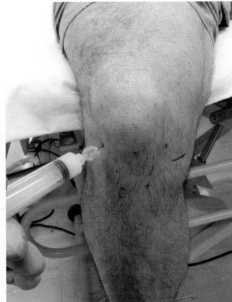

FIGURE
6-4

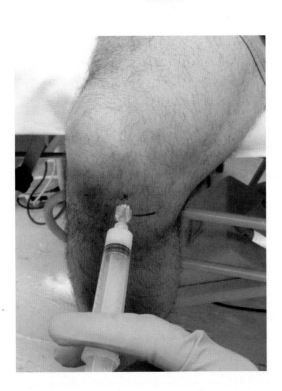

FIGURE
6-5

■ Entry into the joint may be facilitated by eversion (superolateral approach) or inversion (superomedial approach) of the patella.

■ If fluid is not initially obtained, redirect the needle. The needle must be withdrawn until it is just within the skin before redirection. Changing the angle of the needle by withdrawing it first will simply push tissue around (not change its path) and may even risk damage to surrounding tissue, as the bevel may act like a knife.

■ When an intra-articular knee injection is performed in the setting of an open wound to evaluate for the presence of a traumatic arthrotomy, it is important to visually inspect the wound first. Consider the location and subcutaneous extension of the wound, which can often be extensive. Select an approach furthest from the wound in order to minimize the risk of a false-positive result. False negatives are typically encountered in the setting of a small arthrotomy where sufficient fluid is not used to maximally distend the joint. If blood or serous fluid is actively draining from the wound, consider injecting with a diluted methylene blue solution to enhance visualization of the injected fluid.

CLOSED REDUCTIONS

Knee Dislocation

Indication

Any dislocation of the knee is a potentially limb-threatening injury that must be reduced as soon as possible. The posterolateral knee dislocation may be irreducible by closed means due to puncture of the medial capsule by the medial femoral condyle.

Description of Procedure

■ Closed reduction of a true dislocation usually requires conscious sedation or general anesthesia.

■ The knee can dislocate in any direction. However, all closed reductions start with longitudinal traction followed by manipulation of the tibia.

■ Apply in-line traction (Fig. 6-6).

■ Regardless of the direction of dislocation, reduction should be obtained with direct manipulation of the tibia, rather than the femur. The exception to this recommendation is the anterior dislocation when the distal femur should be lifted after the application of axial traction (Fig. 6-7).

■ Splint the knee in approximately 20° of flexion to allow for relaxation of tension on the posterior neurovascular structures. Most knee immobilizers have some flexion built in and therefore can be used as an alternative.

■ Obtain urgent postreduction radiographs to assess reduction.

Tips and Other Considerations

■ Medial dimpling in the setting of the posterolateral knee dislocation signifies piercing of the medial capsule and indicates that a closed reduction may be impossible. However, a closed reduction should still be attempted.

■ Detailed pre- and postreduction neurovascular examinations are critical. Even in the presence of palpable pedal pulses, an ankle–brachial index should still be obtained. An ankle–brachial index of less than 0.9 requires further investigation.

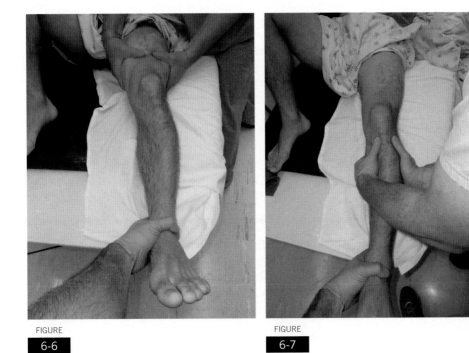

FIGURE
6-6

FIGURE
6-7

- Vascular compromise requires emergent surgical intervention.
- With an intact vascular examination, controversy remains regarding recommendations for traditional angiography versus computed tomography angiography versus serial examinations.

Patellar Dislocations

Indication

The patella nearly always dislocates laterally. Reduction with immobilization in extension can be the definitive treatment of a first-time dislocation without associated injuries if an anatomic reduction is achieved. Recurrent dislocations, those with associated injuries, or irreducible dislocations are often treated operatively; however, reduction is still important to minimize soft tissue and cartilage injury.

Description of Procedure

- In the position of greatest comfort, perform an aspiration of the invariably present hemarthrosis and inject 5 to 10 mL of local anesthetic (see "Intra-articular Knee Injection/ Aspiration"). Aspiration of the hemarthrosis will decompress the knee and facilitate reduction by allowing the patella to lie within the trochlear groove.
- Place the knee in extension. Extension of the knee typically results in the most stable position of the patellofemoral joint. Additionally, knee extension relaxes the extensor mechanism if a reduction is required.

- Often, extension alone will cause reduction of the patella. If not, apply a medially directed force to the laterally dislocated patella.
- Occasionally, slight flexion (approximately 30°) will be required to maintain the reduction since this allows the patella to sit in the deepest portion of the trochlea.
- Immobilize the patient with a brace or cast in the position of the greatest stability.

Tips and Other Considerations

- Rarely, reduction can be achieved but not maintained with positioning alone. In this setting, apply a long leg or cylinder cast (see "Splinting and Casting" section) with a lateral mold over the patella to maintain the reduction.

Tibial Shaft Fractures

Indication

Minimally displaced tibial shaft fractures with length stability can be treated conservatively with a closed reduction and splinting or casting. Most significantly displaced tibial shaft fractures will ultimately require operative treatment; however, closed reduction is still important for avoiding soft tissue and neurovascular complications and pain control.

Tolerances

- Varus/valgus angulation < 5° to 10°.
- Anterior/posterior angulation < 5° to 10°.
- Translation < 50%.
- Shortening < 2 cm.

Description of Procedure

- Assess the deforming forces by evaluating the radiographs. Most commonly, a fracture will usually redisplace to the position of initial displacement. There are, however, some other tendencies.
  - Proximal fractures tend to angulate in valgus and flexion.
  - Isolated fractures of the tibia with an intact fibula usually displace into varus.
  - Tibia fractures with an associated fibula fracture, particularly at the same level, usually displace into valgus.
- Obtain an assistant. Managing the lower limb while simultaneously applying a splint or a cast is extremely difficult.
- Position the patient at the edge of the bed ipsilateral to the injury to allow the leg and part of the thigh to hang off the bed. This position flexes the knee and plantarflexes the ankle, which reduces the most powerful deforming forces (Fig. 6-8).
- Apply traction in-line with the tibia to correct shortening and angular displacement (Fig. 6-9).
- If necessary, apply a rotational correction to align the tibial tubercle and foot in the same relationship as the noninjured side.
- Hold the limb provisionally while the assistant applies a short leg cast.
- Apply a 3-point mold to counteract the deforming forces. Focus on the plane with the most significant angular deformity. Plantar flexion of the ankle will cause a posterior

angulation force, while dorsiflexion of the ankle causes anterior angulation and shortening (Fig. 6-10).

- Now, correct any rotational deformity and extend the cast to the thigh (long leg cast) to lock in the correct rotation.

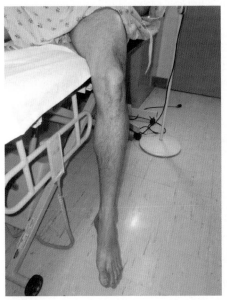

FIGURE
6-8

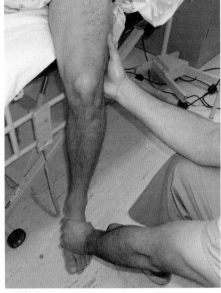

FIGURE
6-9

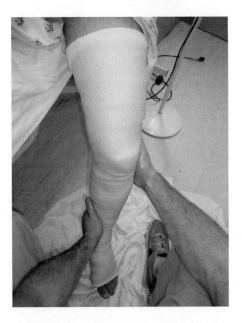

FIGURE
6-10

Tips and Other Considerations

- If there is concern about soft tissue swelling, then the patient should be splinted first, followed by casting after swelling has stabilized (typically 1 to 2 days).
- All attempts to obtain an assistant should be made. If it is not possible, consider applying a short leg cast or splint first and extending it to a long leg cast or splint after it has set and an appropriate mold has been applied.
- In markedly displaced fractures, a provisional reduction and splinting is performed before surgical treatment. In the vast majority of tibial shaft fractures, the anteromedial skin is most at risk; therefore, an intentional malreduction into varus and apex posterior (recurvatum) is performed to take tension off the most compromised soft tissues (Fig. 6-11).

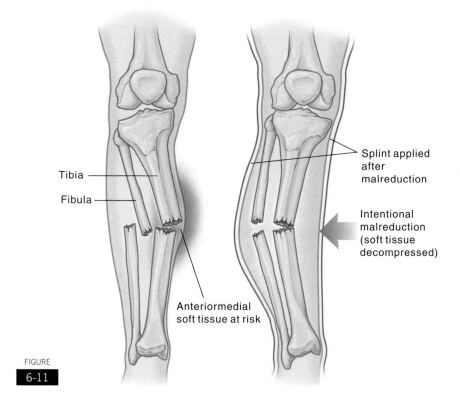

Tibia

Fibula

Splint applied after malreduction

Intentional malreduction (soft tissue decompressed)

Anteriormedial soft tissue at risk

FIGURE
6-11

PROCEDURES

Skeletal Traction

Indication

Skeletal traction is occasionally used in the initial stages of management of acetabular and femoral fractures to facilitate temporary reduction and stabilization before and during operative fixation. It is very rarely used as a definitive treatment modality.

Distal Femoral Traction Pin

Description of Procedure

- The proximal femoral traction pin is placed from medial to lateral to minimize the risk of injury to the femoral artery because the physician has more control at the entry site.
- Position the knee and hip in the amount of flexion that will be present while traction is applied. This step will minimize the pull of the illiotibial band on the pin that will occur with any change in position after it is pierced during pin insertion. Omission of this step may cause unnecessary pain and difficulty positioning the limb.
- Prepare a wide area of the skin with antibacterial solution.
- Anesthetize the skin, subcutaneous tissue, and periosteum on the medial and lateral aspects of the thigh at the level of anticipated pin placement.
- Palpate the adductor tubercle. The entry site will be one fingerbreadth proximal to this landmark. A more proximal starting point increases the risk of damage to the femoral artery, while a more distal starting point places the pin in weaker bone, and risks entering the knee joint or intercondylar notch. Pins in the distal femur are always inserted medial to lateral to minimize the risk of injury to the femoral artery (Fig. 6-12).
- Make a small, longitudinal stab incision through the skin just proximal to the adductor tubercle between the anterior and posterior margins of the femur.
- Use a small clamp to bluntly dissect the femur (Fig. 6-13).
- Insert a 5-mm Steinman pin into the wound. Although we prefer smooth pins because they are stronger; however, a threaded pin can also be used.
- Carefully use the tip of the pin to feel the anterior and posterior margins of the femur and identify the center of the femur.

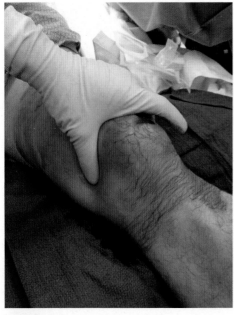

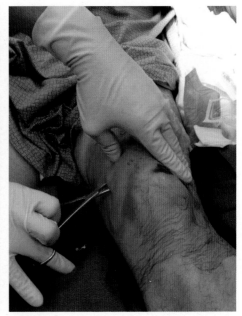

FIGURE
6-12

FIGURE
6-13

- Once you are confident that the pin is centered on the femur, use a hand or power drill to drive the pin through the medial and lateral cortices of the femur.
- When the pin is prominent laterally, make a small, longitudinal stab incision through the skin. A transverse stab incision through the illiotibial band can also be made if necessary. Continue driving the pin until equal amounts are visible on each side of the limb (Figs. 6-14 and 6-15).
- Use a large pin cutter to remove the sharp end of the pin.
- Dress the pin sites, and obtain orthogonal radiographic views before application of traction (Fig. 6-16).

Tips and Other Considerations

- Always perform a physical exam to evaluate the knee for injury. If there is any question, obtain knee radiographs before the procedure to rule out injury in the intended location of pin placement.
- Intravenous narcotics or mild or conscious sedation may be used for additional analgesia/anesthesia; however, successful pin placement can be accomplished with local anesthetic alone.
- Fluoroscopy is not needed to place the traction pin.
- Distal femoral traction pins are typically used in the setting of acetabular fractures. In this case, pin placement parallel to the knee joint line is recommended because it will place the traction force vector closer to and parallel with the mechanical axis of the femur.
- In the setting of femoral shaft fractures, proximal tibial traction pins are more commonly used to avoid interference with eventual hardware placement. However, if a distal femoral

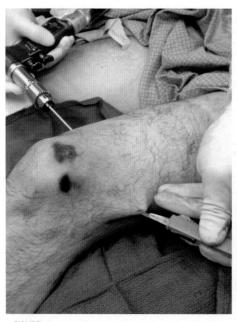

FIGURE
6-14

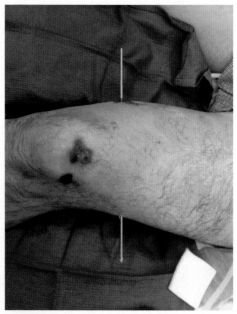

FIGURE
6-15

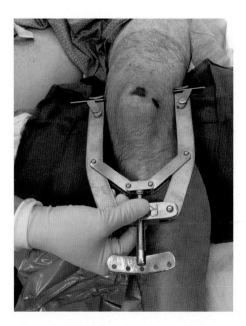

FIGURE
6-16

traction pin is used, pin placement perpendicular to the shaft of the femur is recommended because it will place the traction force vector parallel to the anatomic axis of the femur.

■ After placing the limb in traction ensure that the traction bow does not contact the anterior tibia. Even a very well padded traction bow can cause soft tissue problems (Figs. 6-17 and 6-18).

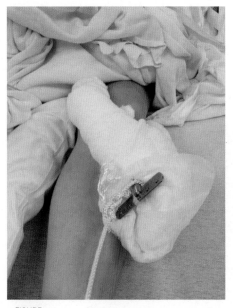

FIGURE
6-17

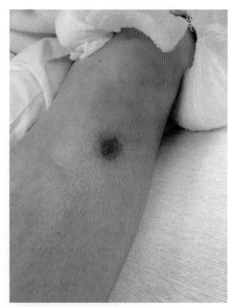

FIGURE
6-18

Proximal Tibial Traction Pin

Description of Procedure

- The proximal tibial traction pin is placed from lateral to medial to minimize the risk of injury to the peroneal nerve because the physician has more control at the entry site.
- Prepare a wide area of the skin with antibacterial solution.
- Anesthetize the skin, subcutaneous tissue, and periosteum on the medial and lateral aspects of the leg at the level of anticipated pin placement.
- Palpate the tibial tubercle. The entry site is approximately 2 cm (about one fingerbreadth) distal and posterior to the tibial tubercle on the lateral aspect of the tibia. More distal pin insertion risks injury to the peroneal nerve (Figs. 6-19 and 6-20).
- Make a small, longitudinal stab incision through the skin at this level (Fig. 6-21).
- Use a small clamp to bluntly dissect the tibia.
- Insert a 4- or 5-mm Steinman pin into the wound.
- Position the pin centrally on the lateral cortex by feeling the anterior and posterior margins of the tibia.
- Use a hand or power drill to drive the pin through the lateral and medial cortices of the tibia.
- When the pin is prominent medially, make a small, longitudinal stab incision through the skin, and continue driving the pin until equal amounts are visible on each side of the limb (Fig. 6-22).
- Use a large pin cutter to remove the sharp end of the pin.
- Dress the pin sites and obtain orthogonal radiographic views before application of traction (Fig. 6-23).

Tips and Other Considerations

- Always perform a physical exam to evaluate the knee for injury. If there is any question, obtain knee radiographs before the procedure to rule out injury in the intended location of pin placement.
- The most common error is to place the skin incision too anterior. This results in either an anterior pin or soft tissue stretch if the pin is central on the tibia.

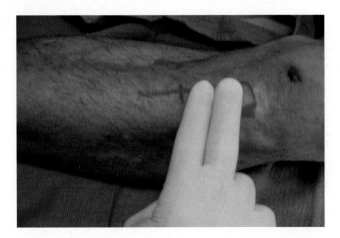

FIGURE

6-19

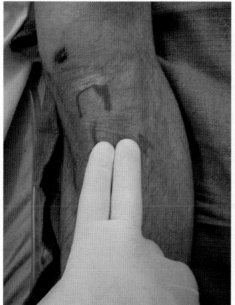

FIGURE
6-20

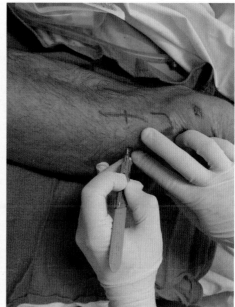

FIGURE
6-21

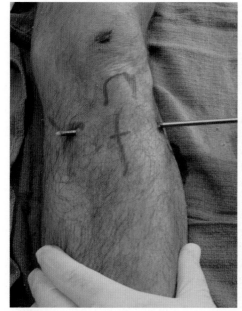

FIGURE
6-22

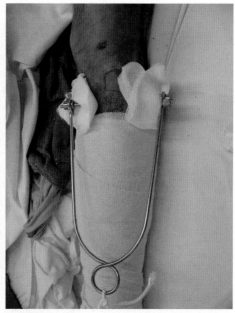

FIGURE
6-23

- Avoid prolonged skeletal traction through a proximal tibial traction in children with open physes.
- Intravenous narcotics or mild or conscious sedation may be used for additional analgesia/anesthesia; however, successful pin placement can be accomplished with local anesthetic alone.
- Fluoroscopy is not needed to place the traction pin.
- In small children, an alternative to skeletal traction is skin traction. Weight should not exceed 5 to 10 lb to avoid injury to the skin. Periodic examination of the skin is necessary.

Compartment Pressure Measurement in the Leg

Indication

Compartment syndrome occurs when the pressure within the fascial compartment exceeds capillary pressure, leading to tissue ischemia. It is an orthopaedic emergency and requires emergent fasciotomy. The use of compartment pressure measurement in the diagnosis of compartment syndrome is controversial. Because false negatives and false positives can occur, pressure measurements can fluctuate with time and proximity to the traumatized tissue, and the pressure that defines compartment syndrome is unknown, we prefer to make the diagnosis on the basis of clinical examination when possible. Compartment pressure measurement is utilized when the patient is intoxicated, obtunded, or otherwise incapable of cooperating with an examination. When performed, we define compartment syndrome when the compartment pressure is within 30 mm Hg of the patient's diastolic blood pressure.

Description of Procedure

- The leg contains four compartments: anterior, lateral, superficial posterior, and deep posterior (Fig. 6-24).
- Position the patient supine.
- Prepare a wide area of the skin with antibacterial solution.
- *Optional*: Mark the entry site with a marking pen. Perform this step before application of antibacterial solution, if a nonsterile pen is used.
- Three entry sites are required to access the four compartments of the leg. Although the preferred level for pressure measurement varies based upon the injury, the junction of the proximal and middle thirds of the leg/tibia is ideal because many of the muscles become tendinous distally.
  - Anterior Compartment: The entry site is located between the easily palpable crest of the tibia and intermuscular septum between the lateral and anterior compartments (Fig. 6-25).
  - Lateral Compartment: The entry site is 1 cm lateral to the palpable intermuscular septum between the anterior and lateral compartments (Fig. 6-26).
  - Posterior Compartments: The tibia is relatively triangular shaped, and the medial aspect is subcutaneous. The entry site is located approximately two fingerbreadths posterior to the palpable posteromedial corner of the tibia (Figs. 6-27 and 6-28).
- *Optional*: Anesthetize the skin overlying the planned entry site with 2 to 3 mL of local anesthetic.
- Assemble the intracompartmental pressure-measuring device according to the manufacturer's specifications. Alternatively, an arterial line system with high-pressure tubing and a wick catheter can be used.

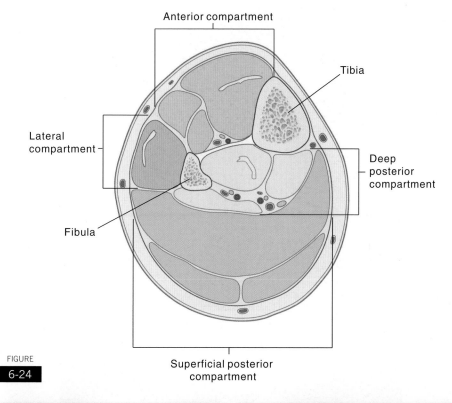

Anterior compartment

Tibia

Lateral compartment

Deep posterior compartment

Fibula

Superficial posterior compartment

FIGURE
6-24

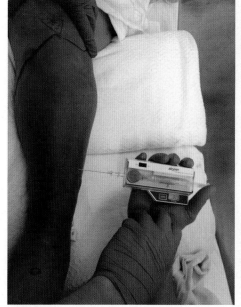

FIGURE
6-25

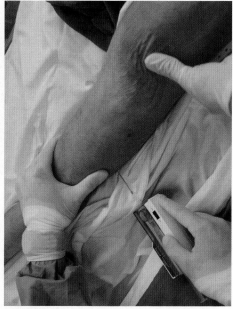

FIGURE
6-26

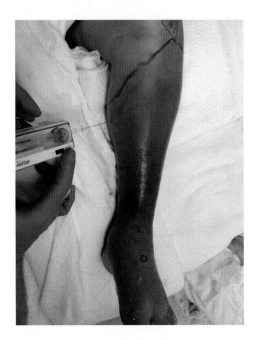

FIGURE
6-27

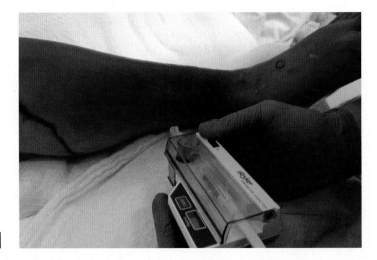

FIGURE
6-28

■ Hold the needle/pressure transducer at the level of the entry site and at the angle of insertion. For each compartment, the angle will be such that the needle is directed centrally (toward the tibia).

■ Zero the system.

■ For the anterior, lateral, and superficial posterior compartments, insert the needle approximately 3 cm. For the deep posterior compartment, advance the needle further. If a pressure difference is not observed as the needle moves from the superficial to deep posterior compartment, advance the needle until it comes into contact with the posterior aspect of the tibia. Now angle the needle slightly posterior, guaranteeing that the needle is in the deep posterior compartment.

Tips and Other Considerations

- Immediately after needle insertion, it is common for the pressure reading to become temporarily elevated before trending down and stabilizing at a value. Ensure enough passage of time to record a stable value, and avoid recording the initial, potentially falsely elevated value.
- For greatest accuracy, we recommend assessing the mean of three separate measurements in each compartment.
- An assistant should write down the pressures for each compartment as you call them out.

PEDIATRIC CONSIDERATIONS

Physeal Injury: Distal Femur

Indication

Nondisplaced distal femur physeal injuries can be treated nonoperatively in a long leg or hip spica cast (depending on the patient's anatomy). Displaced fractures are treated operatively because an anatomic reduction is required; however, an atraumatic, closed reduction is important for minimizing the extent of the injury to the physis and soft tissues.

Description of Procedure

- Perform a carful neurovascular exam. In particular, displacement in the sagittal plane can be associated with an injury to the neurovascular structures in the popliteal fossa, similar to other injuries around the knee.
- As with any fracture involving the physis, it is important for the reduction to be as atraumatic as possible. For this reason, we typically perform a reduction of a distal femur physeal fracture under conscious sedation in the Emergency Department or general anesthesia in the operating room (before operative treatment).
- Apply constant traction by placing both hands around the ankle or tibia. Traction is the single most important maneuver for reduction. It is important to apply sufficient traction to allow for atraumatic manipulation of the physis without iatrogenic injury.
- The second step involves correction of the angular deformity. Some will typically already have been corrected by traction alone. Correct the remainder utilizing some degree of knee flexion; fractures with anterior displacement require more than those with posterior displacement.
- Finally, apply some gentle manipulation to counteract the translational displacement.
- Maintain traction while a long leg splint or cast (see "Splinting and Casting" section) is applied.
- After the splint or cast has been applied, allow your assistant to maintain traction while you apply the appropriate mold.

Tips and Other Considerations

- A fluoroscopy unit can be extremely helpful as it may be difficult to assess the quality of the reduction clinically due to soft tissue edema.

Physeal Injury: Proximal Tibia

Indication

Salter–Harris I and II fractures of the proximal tibia can often be treated nonoperatively if an anatomic reduction is obtained. For injuries involving the articular surface, displacement typically necessitates surgical treatment. An atraumatic, closed reduction can still be helpful for minimizing the extent of the injury to the physis and soft tissues.

Description of Procedure

- Perform a careful neurovascular exam. In particular, displacement in the sagittal plane can be associated with an injury to the neurovascular structures in the popliteal fossa, similar to other injuries around the knee. Proximal tibial fractures, in particular, have a relatively high rate of compartment syndrome.
- The major deforming force is the extensor mechanism of the knee, as the patellar tendon inserts on the tibial tubercle.
- As with any fracture involving the physis, it is important for the reduction to be as atraumatic as possible. For this reason, we typically perform a reduction of a proximal tibial physeal fracture under conscious sedation in the Emergency Department or general anesthesia in the operating room (before operative treatment).
- Apply constant traction by placing both hands around the ankle or tibia. Traction is the single most important maneuver for reduction. It is important to apply sufficient traction to allow for atraumatic manipulation of the physis without iatrogenic injury.
- Extend the knee while maintaining traction.
- If available, use your fluoroscopy unit to evaluate the reduction. Many fractures are reduced at this point in the procedure.
- If necessary, apply gentle manipulation to counteract deforming forces while an assistant maintains traction. Typically, this is necessary if the distal fragment is posteriorly translated. To reduce this displacement, apply a posteriorly directed force proximal to the fracture and an anteriorly directed force distal to the fracture.
- Coronal plane deformity is less common. If present, address last by applying a varus or valgus force while the knee is in extension.
- Once reduced, maintain gentle traction with the knee slightly flexed (10° to 15°) while an assistant applies a splint (see "Splinting and Casting" section).

Tips and Other Considerations

- A fluoroscopy unit can be extremely helpful as it may be difficult to assess the quality of the reduction due to soft tissue.
- Because of the displacement pattern, the anterior tibial artery may become stretched and/or injured leading to a relatively high rate of compartment syndrome. If a reduction is performed, admission and close observation for 24 hours should be considered. A splint is preferred to a cast in the acute setting. If the patient is treated nonoperatively, the splint can be exchanged for a cast after 3 to 7 days.

FIGURE CREDITS

Figure 6-17   Courtesy of Conor Kleweno M.D
Figure 6-18   Courtesy of Conor Kleweno M.D

The Ankle

INJECTIONS AND ASPIRATIONS

Intra-articular Ankle Injection and Aspiration: Antero-medial and Antero-lateral

Indication

Intra-articular positioning of a needle provides the physician with the ability to obtain synovial fluid for analysis (e.g., to differentiate gout vs. septic arthritis), provide local anesthesia for procedures, evaluate for traumatic arthrotomy, and treat degenerative conditions with a variety of medicines.

Description of Procedure

- Position the patient upright with the ankle dependent with gravity. The use of gravity helps manually distract the joint. If needed, an assistant can "pull" the ankle as well, but usually this is not needed.
- Prepare a wide area of the skin with antibacterial solution.
- The ankle and foot lend themselves to careful palpation, given theirs subcutaneous location.
- The perfect spot for an ankle injection is just medial to the anterior tibialis tendon at the level of the joint line. The joint line can usually be palpated by running your thumb on the anterior aspect of the distal tibia until a soft spot is felt as the thumb enters into the joint line (Fig. 7-1).
- An anterolateral injection can be used as well. It is slightly more difficult than the antero-medial injection but useful for cases with medial cellulitis or traumatic wounds. There is a soft spot just lateral to the EDL tendon that is the ideal spot for anterolateral injections. The main area of concern is the superficial peroneal nerve, which is to be avoided. (See section on ankle blocks.)
- *Optional:* Anesthetize the skin overlying the planned entry site with 2 to 3 mL of local anesthetic. However, if an infection is being ruled out, do not use local anesthesia as lidocaine can act as a bacteriostatic agent and decrease the chance of a positive culture.
- Direct the needle through the skin into the ankle joint. We typically use a 22G needle for injections. If bone is encountered, either raise or lower your hand as the needle is hitting either distal tibia or talus.
- Aspirate synovial fluid to verify that the needle is appropriately positioned. If no fluid is withdrawn, attempt injecting minimally. Often, it is difficult to withdraw fluid from the ankle unless an effusion is present. If there is resistance, stop the injection and consider using a fluoroscopic image machine for assistance.
- Continue aspirating or inject the desired solution.
- Apply a sterile, compressive dressing.

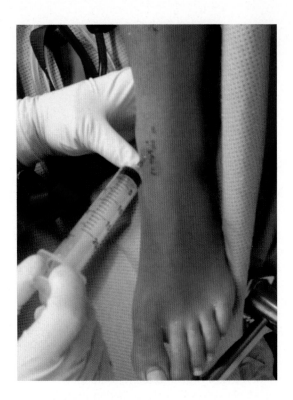

FIGURE

7-1

Tips and Other Considerations

- The use of local anesthetic is debatable. Some physicians feel it is not helpful because only the skin will be anesthetized and a second injection is required. In the pediatric setting, fewer injections are better.

- Entry into the joint may be facilitated by plantarflexing and manually distracting the ankle by wrapping the posterior aspect of the ankle with your nondominant hand and pulling distally.

- If fluid is not initially obtained, redirect the needle. The needle must be withdrawn until it is just within the skin before redirection. Changing the angle of the needle without withdrawing it first will simply push tissue around (not change its path) and may even risk damage to surrounding tissue, as the bevel may act like a knife.

- A typical mistake is inserting the needle too proximal making it impossible to enter the joint.

- When an intra-articular ankle injection is performed in the setting of a fracture, usually a large effusion is present and it is difficult to feel the joint line. In this setting, however, the use of local anesthesia can be very helpful in performing closed reductions of displaced or dislocated ankle fractures. Often, we use a large-bore needle (18G) to "find" the effusion and withdraw some of the blood and then switch syringes to fill the joint with local anesthetic. This procedure usually provides the patient a significant decrease in pain for the attempted closed reduction.

Regional Ankle Block

Indication

A regional ankle block is a useful procedure to produce local anesthesia for the entire foot. We find it especially helpful for exploring the plantar surface of the foot for a foreign body or for a plantar debridement. It may be used for anesthesia for a variety of outpatient foot procedures as well.

Description of Procedure

- Position the patient in a supine position with the knee extended; external rotation at the hip will help gain access to the medial side of the ankle.
- Prepare a wide area of the skin with antibacterial solution.
- We prefer to inject the local solution with a 22G needle. An 18G needle seems to be too large and can cause too much damage, while a 25G needle can make the infusion of a large volume of fluid very difficult.
- We typically use a mixture of 1% lidocaine and 0.5% Marcaine, both without epinephrine, mixed in a one to one ratio.
- Depending on the area of the foot that the provider wishes to anesthetize, one or more of the following nerves may be anesthetized.
  - Tibial nerve for the plantar foot.
  - Superficial and deep peroneal nerves for the dorsum of the foot. The deep peroneal nerve supplies sensation to the first web space.
  - Saphenous nerve for the medial hindfoot and midfoot.
  - Sural nerve for the lateral foot.

Posterior Tibial Nerve Block

- The use of a 4-inch Esmarch bandage tourniquet in the supra-malleolar region before the injection can produce a temporary distal ischemia, which will potentiate the effects of the local anesthesia. We will try to keep the Esmarch bandage on for 3 to 5 minutes after the injection is given.
- The critical spot for an ankle block is just medial to the Achilles tendon at the level of the inferior medial malleolus. This will block the posterior tibial nerve leading to plantar sensory anesthesia.
- The needle is directed toward the medial malleolus, and an effort is made for the needle to touch the bone. After touching the bone, withdraw the needle 1 mm and inject 10 mL of the solution (Fig. 7-2).
- Ideally, about half the length of the 22G needle should be under the skin when blocking the posterior tibial nerve (Fig. 7-3).

Deep Peroneal Nerve Block

- To block the deep peroneal nerve in the midfoot, palpate the base of the first web interspace just lateral to the extensor hallucis longus (EHL) tendon. The needle is advanced to the underlying tarsal bones and withdrawn 1 to 2 mm for injection. The nerve is lateral to the dorsalis pedis artery.

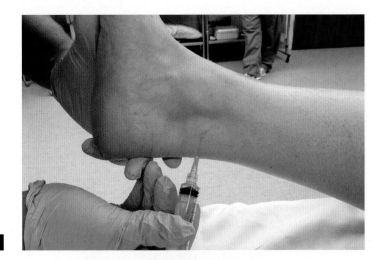

FIGURE
7-2

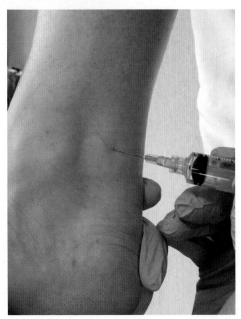

FIGURE
7-3

■ The deep peroneal nerve has a small sensory distribution; therefore, this portion of the block is not needed unless working in the first web space.

Ring Block: Superficial Peroneal, Sural, and Saphenous Nerve Blocks

■ There are two ways to approach this block. The first is to locate each nerve by using the anatomic location and inject only in that area. The second is to inject a "ring" of local anesthetic in the subcutaneous tissue of the midfoot to anesthetize all dorsal nerves. We prefer the ring block because it is quicker and more effective in anesthetizing the entire dorsum of the foot.

■ It is easy to locate terminal branches of the superficial peroneal nerve in a thin patient by plantarflexing the fourth toe and observing a spaghetti-like fiber or cord on the anterior lateral aspect of the ankle (Fig. 7-4). However, we do not routinely look for these nerve branches. Instead, the ring block is performed by infiltrating local anesthetic in the subcutaneous tissues across the entire dorsum of the foot (Figs. 7-5 and 7-6).

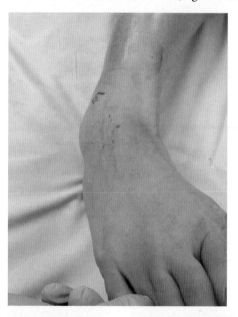

FIGURE
7-4

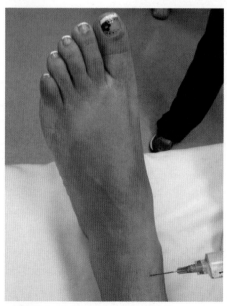

FIGURE
7-5

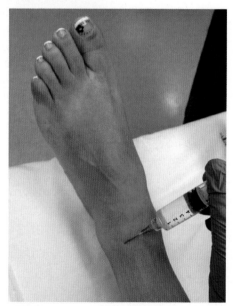

FIGURE
7-6

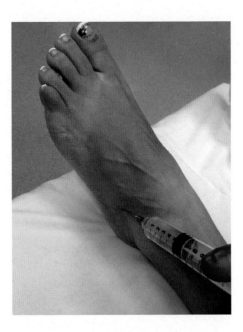

FIGURE

7-7

- The saphenous nerve is blocked by continuing to inject in the subcutaneous tissues on the medial side of the foot down to the glabrous/nonglabrous junction.
- To block the sural nerve, palpate the tip of the distal fibula and continue injection of the ring block until the plantar skin is encountered distal to the fibula (Fig. 7-7).

Tips and Other Considerations

- In an awake patient, when performing the ring block, it is much less painful for the patient to inject in areas that have already been touched subcutaneously with local anesthesia. Therefore, when creating a block, watch as the skin is elevated and then inject in that area. Do not try to obtain access in areas that have not been touched yet by the anesthetic.
- With a proper block of the posterior tibial nerve, you will often see a visual redness to plantar surface of the foot. This is a blockade of the sympathetic fibers resulting in a capillary expansion and subsequent hyperemia.
- The most common error is failure to fully incorporate the most plantar branches of both the saphenous and sural nerves.
- Restrict the patient's weightbearing status after the procedure. The plantar surface of the foot will be numb, and walking and driving are difficult and dangerous.

FRACTURES AND DISLOCATIONS

Reduction of Ankle Fractures and Dislocations

Indication

Ankle fractures are very common. Often, the talus will be displaced laterally or, less commonly, medially. The goal of reduction is to center the talus under the tibia plafond in all planes. Most fractures that require a reduction will mandate an eventual surgical intervention. However, reducing the fracture promptly and correctly will diminish any tension on the skin and prevent propagation of severe soft tissue swelling.

Description of Procedure

- Position the patient supine with the knee flexed over the end of the bed.
- An intra-articular ankle injection can be done with 1% lidocaine to help ease the pain of the reduction. Give the ankle injection time (10 to 15 minutes) to set up.
- Conscious sedation in the emergency room (ER) setting can help in patients with muscular anatomy or widely displaced fractures, but is usually not necessary with a properly placed intra-articular injection.
- The reduction, as usual, involves recreating the mechanism of injury with exaggeration and then the contra-maneuver to reduce the fracture. Most ankle fractures are caused by some element of external rotation. Therefore, the reduction involves internal rotation and supination or pronation combined with distal traction (Fig. 7-8).
- Often, there is an audible or palpable clunk as the talus reduces under the tibia.
- For a patient with a left ankle fracture or dislocation: Place the palm of your left hand against the patient's medial distal tibia and your right hand cupping the lateral aspect of the heel. Next, rotate your right hand with internal rotation, medial translation, and traction to reduce the fracture (Figs. 7-9 through 7-11).

Tips and Other Considerations

- A simple trick in ankle reductions involves grasping the great toe and lifting the limb. If the patient is supine with the leg in external rotation, this will lead to internal rotation, supination, and adduction—the necessary maneuver for the reduction. Adequate relaxation is necessary for this to occur. The use of finger traps on the great toe is also an option for this maneuver, and it allows the application of a splint without an assistant (Fig. 7-12).

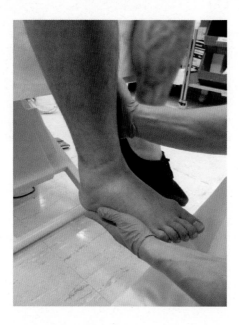

FIGURE

7-8

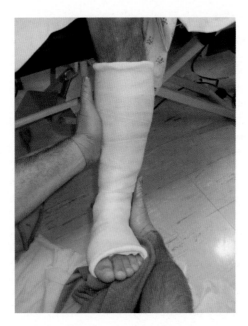

FIGURE

7-9

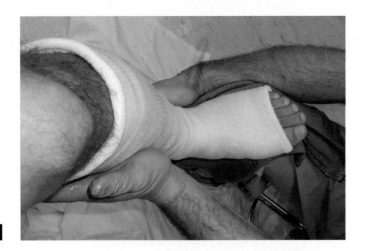

FIGURE

7-10

- The goal of reduction is an anatomic reduction of the ankle mortise. If this is not accomplished, another attempt should be made.
- Good splinting techniques are essential to maintain the reduction. A well-molded U-splint is an excellent choice to maintain the reduction. A short leg cast can also be placed, but if a reduction is performed the cast should be bivalved to allow for swelling.

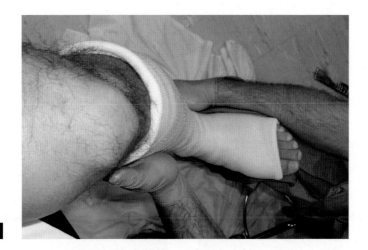

FIGURE
7-11

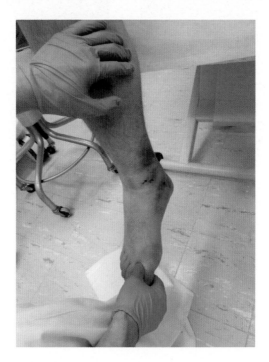

FIGURE
7-12

■ Equinus positioning of the leg should be avoided because it is a nonfunctional position and increases rotational instability. Occasionally, some degree of equinus is desired to keep the ankle from dislocating posteriorly. In these cases, equinus positioning is desirable to leaving the ankle subluxated or dislocated.

■ The only mechanism where the talus displaces medially involves a supination–adduction (SAD) type of mechanism (Fig. 7-13). These are the least likely of ankle fractures to occur. In these special cases, the reduction maneuver is the opposite. Lateral translation of the talus is achieved by everting the heel with a laterally directed force. If a SAD ankle fracture reduction is approached the same way as the more common lateral dislocated ankle, then you will actually worsen the deformity (Fig 7-14).

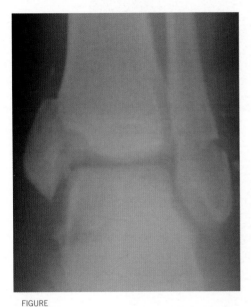

FIGURE
7-13

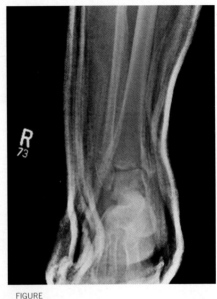

FIGURE
7-14

The Foot

INJECTIONS AND ASPIRATIONS

Plantar Fascia Injection

Indication

Plantar fascia injections are used for the treatment of plantar fasciitis. They are commonly performed in the outpatient setting and are used once initial conservative measures to control the fasciitis have failed.

Description of Procedure

- Position the patient upright with the ankle dependent with gravity.
- Prepare a wide area of the skin with antibacterial solution.
- The ankle and foot lend themselves to careful palpation, given their subcutaneous location.
- The perfect spot for the plantar fascia injection is in-line with the posterior aspect of the medial malleolus extended distally to the level of the skin transition to the glabrous skin from the plantar side of the foot (Fig. 8-1).
- *Optional*: Anesthetize the skin overlying the planned entry site with 2 to 3 mL of local anesthetic. However, this is a relatively painful and sensitive area of the skin, and we would warn against this.

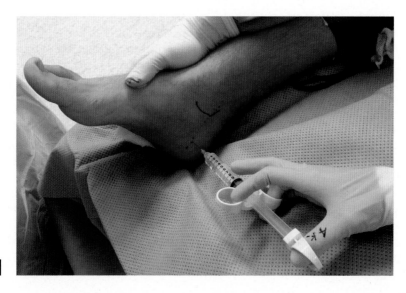

FIGURE
8-1

- Direct the needle through the medial skin and toward the calcaneus. We typically use a 22G or 25G needle for injections. Once bone is encountered, withdraw the needle slightly and raise your hand to plantarly direct the needle into the fascia origin area.
- Apply a sterile, compressive dressing or a adhesive dressing after any initial bleeding is stopped with direct pressure.

Tips and Other Considerations

- A plantar approach for this injection has been described, but we find it excessively painful for the patient and do not use it.
- The topical use of an ethylene chloride spray can minimize the discomfort of this injection. If using a 25G needle, be careful not to spray and freeze the needle making the injection even more difficult.
- We typically use 1 cc of lidocaine 1% plain mixed with 1 cc of a steroid of your choosing. Usually, we use either depomedrol 40 mg/ml or Kenalog 10 mg/ml. 0.5% plain Marcaine can be added as well, but it can lengthen the duration of the injection.
- This injection is among the most difficult to perform.
- This is usually a second-tier option for the treatment of plantar fasciitis. Initially, we try plantar fascia-specific stretching, nonsteroidal anti-inflammatory drug (NSAIDs), physical therapy, and night splints. After the above have failed to relieve the pain for 4 to 6 weeks, an injection is indicated.

Subtalar Joint Injection and Aspiration: Sinus Tarsi Approach

Indication

The sinus tarsi is a conical space on the lateral ankle that provides a window to the subtalar joint. Injections can be given to help with synovitis, arthritis, and for diagnostic purposes.

Description of Procedure

- Position the patient sitting with the leg internally rotated.
- Inverting the ankle can help to "open" the sinus tarsi.
- Alternatively, the use of gravity helps manually distract the joint. If needed, an assistant can "pull" the ankle as well, but usually this is not needed.
- Prepare a wide area of the skin with antibacterial solution.
- The ankle and foot then themselves to careful palpation, given their subcutaneous location.
- The perfect spot for a sinus tarsi injection is just anterior to the distal tip of the fibula, usually about two fingerbreadths anteriorly. The sinus tarsi can usually be palpated by running your thumb toward the toes from the anterior aspect of the distal fibula until a soft spot is felt as the thumb enters into the sinus tarsi (Fig. 8-2).
- *Optional:* Anesthetize the skin overlying the planned entry site with 2 to 3 mL of local anesthetic. However, if an infection is being ruled out, do not use local anesthesia as lidocaine can act as a bacteriostatic agent and decrease the chance of a positive culture.
- Direct the needle superiorly and posteriorly through the skin into the sinus tarsi. We typically use a 22G needle for injections. If bone is encountered, either raise or lower

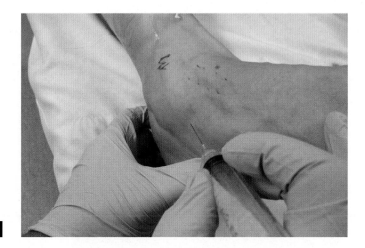

FIGURE
8-2

your hand as the needle is hitting either dorsal calcaneus or plantar talus. Usually, the error is to be too superior, so raising your hand will lower the needle into the tarsi.
- Aspirate synovial fluid to verify that the needle is appropriately positioned. If no fluid is withdrawn, attempt injecting minimally. Often, it is difficult to withdraw fluid from the sinus tarsi unless an effusion is present. If there is resistance, stop the injection and consider using a fluoroscopic image machine for assistance.
- Continue aspirating or inject the desired solution.
- Apply a sterile, compressive dressing.

Tips and Other Considerations

- The use of local anesthetic is debatable. Some physicians feel it is not helpful because only the skin will be anesthetized and a second injection is required. In the pediatric setting, the fewer injections given the better.
- Entry into the joint may be facilitated by plantarflexing and inverting the ankle.
- If fluid is not initially obtained, redirect the needle. The needle must be withdrawn until it is just within the skin before redirection. Changing the angle of the needle without withdrawing it first will simply push tissue around (not change its path) and may even risk damage to surrounding tissue, as the bevel may act like a knife.
- This is among the most difficult injections to perform.
- If available, the use of fluoroscopy is very helpful. A radiographic marker is placed on the proposed insertion side, and a lateral fluoroscopic image is taken to confirm the correct insertion point. If the mark is incorrectly placed, then move it until it is directly over the sinus tarsi.
- Using fluoroscopy, the subtalar joint can also be approached from posterior to enter the joint at the larger posterior facet.
  - In the lateral position, place the needle just anterior to the lateral aspect of the Achilles tendon. Using the fluoroscopy unit, direct the needle into the posterior facet of the subtalar joint. You will feel a slight "pop" as the needle pierces the joint capsule. Confirm the position with the fluoroscopy and inject as desired (Fig. 8-3).

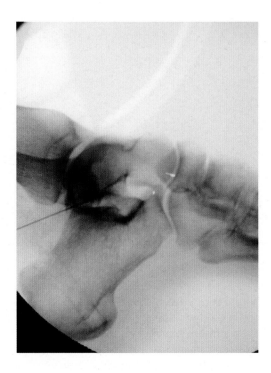

FIGURE
8-3

Digital Toe Block

Indication

A toe block is a useful procedure to produce local anesthesia for an entire toe. We find it especially helpful for reducing proximal phalanx fractures and, more commonly, nail plate removals. It is often used before many outpatient foot and toe procedures as well.

Description of Procedure

- Position the patient in a supine position with the knee extended.
- Prepare a wide area of the skin with antibacterial solution at the base of the affected toe.
- We prefer to inject the local solution with a 25G needle. An 18G or 22G needle seems to be too large and can cause too much damage. A 22G needle is used when difficulty injecting the fluid is encountered.
- We typically use 1% or 2% lidocaine. To help with postprocedure pain, 0.5% Marcaine can be added later, but it takes longer to work and can delay the onset of the procedure.
- Never use epinephrine, as it is felt to increase the risk of digital ischemia.
- The digital nerves to the toes are found at the medial and lateral base of the toe of interest. Two different injections should be given: one medially and one laterally
  - Initially, a wheal is raised medial or lateral. Next, through the wheal, the needle is advanced in dorsal and plantar direction. The most common error is to not place the needle planter enough. Finally, the needle is turned horizontally and the dorsum of

the toe is blocked. If needed, the needle can be advanced out the plantar skin to ensure the block is plantar enough.

Tips and Other Considerations

■ Make sure to give the block enough time to work. We find it helpful to place the block, complete other tasks and paperwork, and return to the patient in 10 to 15 minutes. One of the main failures and causes of pain for patients is not letting the block set up adequately.

■ In an awake patient, when performing the toe block, it is much less painful for the patient to inject in areas that have already been touched subcutaneously with local anesthesia. Therefore, when creating a block, watch as the skin is elevated (wheal) and then inject in that area. Do not try to obtain access in areas that have not been touched yet by the anesthetic.

■ For the great toe, 4 to 6 mL of 1% lidocaine is typically used for a complete toe block. For the lesser toes, less volume is needed.

FRACTURES AND DISLOCATIONS

Reduction of Tongue-Type Calcaneal Fractures

Indication

Not all calcaneal fractures are equal. While the majority of calcaneal fractures can be splinted with a bulky casts (Jones dressing; see section on splints and dressings), occasionally a tongue-type fracture with posterior displacement represents a surgical emergency. These types of fractures are problematic because they will exert pressure on the posterior skin of the ankle and can lead to full thickness necrosis of skin, which can lead to amputations. Therefore, recognition of this type of fracture is essential and an urgent closed reduction needs to be performed (Fig. 8-4).

Description of Procedure

■ Position the patient prone, if possible. Keep in mind that the majority of calcaneal fractures are not isolated injuries and the energy imparted can lead to other musculoskeletal injuries making prone positioning impractical. If not possible, this can be done in the lateral position as well.

■ Pressure on the posterior heel while plantarflexing the foot may help reduce pressure on the posterior skin.

■ If this does not result in a change in the fracture pattern or displacement, then urgent closed reduction in the operating room with percutaneous fixation should be undertaken.

Tips and Other Considerations

■ An ominous sign for skin compromise is blanching of the skin over the prominent fragment or a hemorrhagic fracture blister on the posterior heel (Fig. 8-5).

■ These are important fractures not to be missed. If the patient is discharged from the emergency room (ER) with these types of fractures, skin damage can be catastrophic.

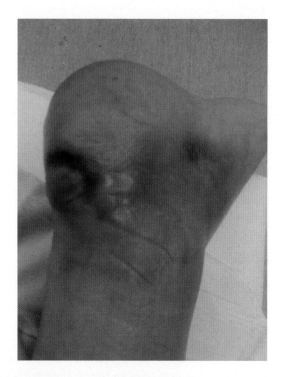

FIGURE
8-4

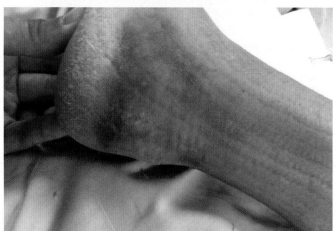

FIGURE
8-5

Evaluation and Reduction of Talar Neck Fractures

Indication

Talar neck fractures represent a significant injury to the foot because they frequently result in long-term disability. Displaced talar neck fractures, particularly when the talar body is dislocated, are emergent issues. If the fracture can be reduced and the overlying soft tissues are decompressed, then the ultimate fixation can be done at a later setting. However, if the fracture cannot be reduced and the ankle or subtalar joint remains dislocated after attempted reduction, urgent surgical open reduction and internal fixation (ORIF) must be undertaken.

Description of Procedure

- Position the patient supine.
- Manipulate the foot into maximal plantar flexion to align the talar head with the rest of the foot.
- Now reduce the subtalar joint with either inversion or eversion depending on whether the subtalar joint is dislocated medially or laterally.
- If not reducible, do not continue with multiple attempts.
- The goal of this reduction is to decrease tension on the skin, not to get a perfect alignment on x-ray.
- The talar body usually rotates posterior and medial around the deep fibers of the posterior deltoid ligament. It is usually impossible to close reduce the talar body, and therefore open reduction is almost always required.

Tips and Other Considerations

- With a displaced talar neck fracture, the overlying contour of the ankle is distorted, and landmarks will be difficult to appreciate.
- Any displaced talus fracture that is causing tension on the skin needs to be emergently closed reduced. This will relieve pressure on the skin and restore more natural circulation to the affected area.
- We do not consider a nondisplaced fracture to be a surgical emergency.
- Keep in mind that talar neck fracture is suspected when ankle x-rays are negative but the patient has ecchymosis and inability to bear weight. Occasionally, a nondisplaced fracture line will be visible on the lateral x-ray.
- Talar neck fractures with an associated talar body dislocation are surgical emergencies because usually the talar body fragment will rotate medially compressing the neurovascular bundle and skin. These types of fractures are virtually impossible to close reduce and will lead to skin necrosis unless emergently reduced (Fig. 8-6).

Reduction of Subtalar Joint Dislocations

Indication

Subtalar joint dislocations represent a dislocation of both the talonavicular and subtalar joints, while the ankle and calcaneal cuboid joints remain reduced. These injuries are an intermediate stage before a complete talar extrusion. Once reduced, subtalar dislocations can often be treated nonoperatively. The vast majority of subtalar dislocations are medial dislocations with the foot (navicular) dislocated medially around a fixed talus. They can occur from both high-energy mechanism and trivial mechanisms such as landing on another person's foot. Occasionally, there will be intervening structures that prohibit a closed reduction.

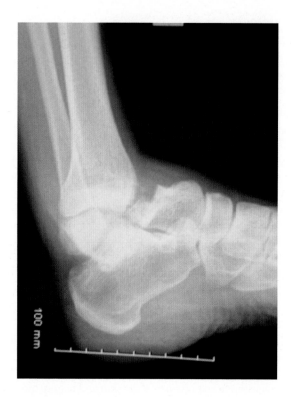

100 mm

FIGURE

8-6

Description of Procedure

- Position the patient upright with the ankle dependent with gravity. If the patient is seen soon after injury, minimal sedation is needed. If not, general or regional anesthesia may be required.
- One essential part of the reduction is flexion of the knee to relax the gastrocnemius–soleus complex. If the patient must remain in a supine position, remember to flex the knee.
- Traction to the heel is applied in all types of subtalar dislocations and if an assistant is available, counter traction at the knee is helpful.
- Direct palpation of the talar head is important, as it will guide the reduction. Essentially, you are trying to guide the dislocated navicular around the talar head.
- Determine whether this is a medial or lateral subtalar dislocation from available radiographs and clinical exam (Fig. 8-7).
- Initially, accentuate the deformity to try to "unlock" it.
  - Medial dislocations: First plantarflex and invert the foot, and then evert, abduct, and dorsiflex the foot. During this time, place medially directed pressure on the laterally displaced talar head with your other hand.
  - Lateral dislocations: First evert the foot to unlock it and then adduct the forefoot. While doing this, place laterally directed force on the medially displaced talar head with your other hand.
- The reduction is often seen, felt, and heard and is not subtle.

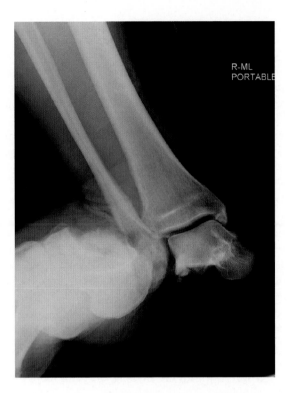

R-ML
PORTABLE

FIGURE
8-7

- Once the subtalar dislocation is reduced, the short leg three-sided splint should be in neutral dorsiflexion and neutral pronation and supination.
- Often, internal fixation is not needed for these injuries, and they can be treated solely with a closed reduction.

Tips and Other Considerations

- Approximately 10% to 20% of the time, a closed reduction will not be possible because of intervening, interposed anatomic structures necessitating an emergent open reduction.
- Remember the knee during the reduction; it is often forgotten and left in extended position, tightening the gastrocnemius, making the reduction unnecessarily difficult.
- While the radiograph may show obvious medial or lateral dislocation, the direction of dislocation is usually obvious by the position of the foot.
- After reduction, a computed tomography (CT) scan should be obtained to check for associated osteochondral fractures, which are common.
- Open injuries are controversial. There is a theoretical risk of increased contamination with ER reductions. However, it is not prudent to leave the foot in a distorted position for a prolonged period of time. If the subtalar dislocation is an isolated injury and an OR is available, then the definite reduction can be done in the OR after a formal irrigation and debridement. If the patient is unstable or has other life-threatening conditions that will delay the orthopaedic operative intervention, then an ER reduction is a good idea.

Evaluation and Reduction of Emergent Midfoot Injuries

Indication

Midfoot and Lisfranc injuries can be from industrial (crush) or high-energy trauma (motor vehicle accidents, falls). Often these patients will present with gross dislocations of the midfoot, severe swelling, and vascular compromise. Emergent reductions can help prevent the propagation of swelling and restoration of vascular flow.

The Lisfranc joint complex is synonymous with the tarsal–metatarsal joint (TMT). The Lisfranc ligament connects the medial cuneiform to the base of the second metatarsal.

Description of Procedure

- An ankle block can be given to diminish the pain experienced by the patient before reduction.
- Overall, longitudinal traction is used at the toes to "pull" the foot out to its proper length. With your other hand, apply gentle pressure to "push" the dislocation back into its normal anatomy. For example, if the first TMT joint was dislocated medially, then longitudinal traction on the great toe followed by laterally directed pressure at the base of the first metatarsal would help reduce the dislocation.
- A palpable or audible clunk is often noted.
- It is essential to carefully evaluate the prereduction radiographs to know exactly where to perform the reduction. Often, the second or third metatarsal will be dislocated dorsally, requiring plantar-directed pressure to reduce it.
- A well-padded splint will help with the swelling and limit motion of the affected foot. Patients need to be completely non–weight bearing.
- These patients should be admitted to the hospital for limb elevation, bed rest, neurovascular monitoring, and possible compartment syndrome.

Tips and Other Considerations

- A handheld Doppler ultrasound unit can help find a dorsalis pedis pulse in the injured, swollen foot. The foot has a rich collateral flow and should always a have a capillary refill of less than two seconds.
- Plantar ecchymosis is an important clinical sign to diagnose a serious midfoot injury. Even if no fractures are present on routine radiographs, be wary of a ligamentous Lisfranc sprain.
- It is easy to be overwhelmed by these injuries because many fractures and dislocations can occur simultaneously. Try to distill the injury into its essential components and focus on the most striking component, which are usually the dislocations (Fig. 8-8).
- There are many Lisfranc "variants" that can occur. Multiple fractures at the bases of the metatarsals should alert the physician that a Lisfranc ligament injury might have occurred as well.
- Closed reduction may not be possible secondary to intervening tendons, bony fragments, and other soft tissue. Do not attempt multiple reductions as this can lead to added chondral and osseous injuries.
- Not all Lisfranc injuries are caused by high-energy trauma and may result from twisting and axial loading. These are so-called Lisfranc "sprains" and demand careful attention, close follow-up, and non–weight-bearing status.

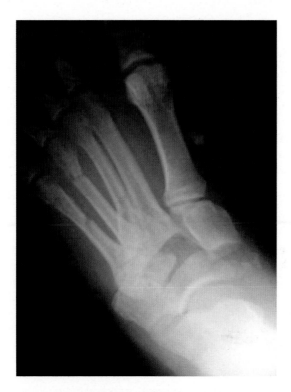

FIGURE
8-8

- Up to 20% of Lisfranc injuries may be missed initially, leading to significant morbidity. Pay careful attention to excessive foot swelling without obvious fractures. Be extremely vigilant with those patients with decreased sensation such as diabetics.
- The so-called "fleck sign" represents an avulsion fracture from either the second MT base or the medial cuneiform. This is due to a forceful abduction of the forefoot that avulses the strong Lisfranc ligament between the base of the second metatarsal and the medial cuneiform.

Evaluation and Treatment of Forefoot Fractures: Closed-Reduction Techniques

Indication

Forefoot fractures are almost always treated closed. Occasionally, a proximal phalanx fracture may be significantly displaced and requires a closed reduction. Most commonly, the fifth toe is involved. The mechanism of injury usually involves walking barefoot at night and impacting the toe against a doorjamb or dresser.

Description of Procedure

- Position the patient supine.
- A toe anesthetic block is usually sufficient (see "toe block"), but be careful not to use too much fluid as this can hamper the reduction. Also perform the toe block more proximal than usual.

- Accentuating the deformity will help with the closed reduction. We usually use a thin-caliber pen or pencil as a fulcrum to reduce the distal toe fracture fragment about. For example, in a fifth toe proximal phalanx fracture with lateral deviation, place the fulcrum in between the fourth and fifth toes (Fig. 8-9).
- After the reduction, tape the toe and the adjacent toe together. If a middle toe is involved, choose the toe to help reduce the prior direction of deformity. For example, if the third toe is displaced laterally, then after the reduction, tape to the second toe to prevent later lateral displacement.
- Use one strand of tape proximally and one strand distally. Paper or cloth tape does not work well, and we prefer plastic tape.

Tips and Other Considerations

- If the fulcrum used for the reduction is too bulky, it will make the reduction more difficult.
- Occasionally, pushing the fulcrum into the webspace positions it optimally for the reduction.
- A post-op rigid shoe is usually given to limit pain after the reduction.
- Patient problems or complaints after a proximal phalanx fracture malunion of the lesser toes have not been a significant problem in our practice. The great toe is less forgiving.
- A thin piece of gauze can be useful between the taped digits to prevent skin maceration.
- A folded piece of gauze can be taped in between two toes to assist in maintaining the reduction.

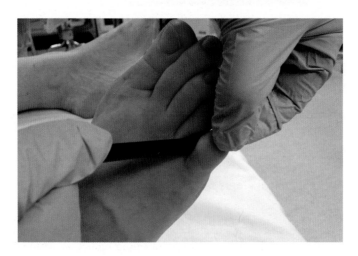

FIGURE
8-9

PROCEDURES

Compartment Pressure Measurement in the Foot

Indication

Compartment syndrome can occur within the foot from severe trauma and postsurgical and various vascular insults. Multistick invasive catheterization is essential for the diagnosis of compartment syndrome and is the most sensitive means available to detect compartment syndrome.

Description of Procedure

- Position the patient supine.
- Avoid local anesthesia as this can mask a nascent compartment syndrome.
- Try to obtain a commercially available pressure monitor; if not available, consult an anesthetist or technologist to help set up an arterial line to monitor the pressure. Multiple catheters have been used to measure compartment pressures. The best catheters have a larger surface area and are less likely to get clogged. Therefore, slit or wick catheters are better than a simple beveled needle.
- Medial compartment pressure is measured 4 cm inferior to the tip of the medial malleolus. Advancing the needle into the abductor hallucis muscle allows measurement of the medial compartment (Fig. 8-10).
- Next, advancing the needle deeper into the calcaneus and slightly withdrawing after touching the medial calcaneus is necessary to measure the calcaneal compartment. (Therefore, both the medial and calcaneal compartment pressures are measured through the same needle trajectory.)
- To measure the superficial compartment, insert the pressure monitor into the superficial, medial arch and penetrate the flexor digitorum brevis. This is best done in the central third of the arch (Fig. 8-11).
- Insertion of the needle inferior to the base of the fifth metatarsal is a good landmark for the measurement of the lateral compartment (Fig. 8-12).
- Separate measurements are made into each of the four interosseous compartments through a dorsal approach. However, if one compartment pressure is significantly elevated, then measuring the rest of the interosseous compartment may not be necessary and can be done in the operating room. Also, advancing the needle deep to one of the interosseous compartments allows measurement of the adductor compartment. We usually use the first or second interosseous space for this. As a general landmark, we try to place the needle 1 to 2 cm proximal to the metatarsal heads for the interosseous compartments.

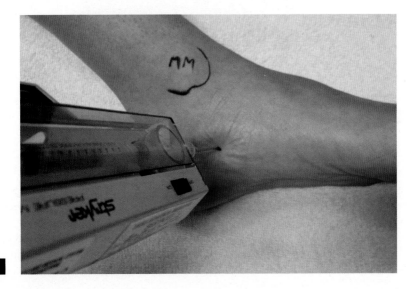

FIGURE
8-10

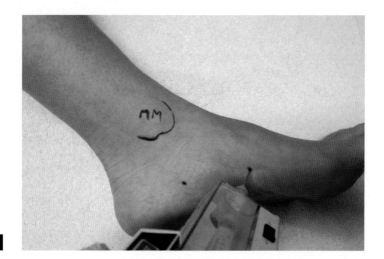

FIGURE
8-11

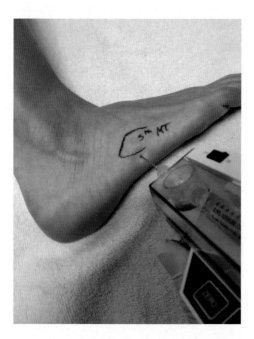

FIGURE
8-12

Tips and Other Considerations

- During actual pressure measurement, the number can vary from minor motion in the examiner's hand. To account for this, try to obtain the number that best represents the average of multiple measurements.
- Have an assistant nearby to write down the compartment pressure measurements.
  - Since there are so many measurements to take, a prewritten outline can help.

- Pain out of proportion to injury is difficult to manage in the presence of calcaneal fractures, crush injuries, or displaced Lisfranc injuries because these injuries are notoriously painful already. If intravenous narcotics are not alleviating the patient's pain significantly, then a compartment syndrome must be considered.
- Open fractures do not necessarily mean the compartment has been released.
- The calcaneal compartment is very small but can cause many problems if missed, make sure the needle tips abut against the bone.
- Make sure to consult with on-call faculty or staff before measuring compartments. If pressure measurements mandate fasciotomy, then the case becomes an emergency. Your attending surgeon will want to know about the patient as early as possible. This is particularly important for residents.
- Fasciotomy is usually performed for pressures above 30 mm Hg or within 10 to 30 mm Hg of diastolic pressure; this is based on research from forearm and leg compartment syndromes.
- Before fasciotomy, elevation of the foot to the level of the heart but not above is prudent. Further elevation may reduce inflow to an already compromised tissue.
- Long-term sequelae of an unrecognized compartment syndrome of the foot can include claw toe deformities, weakness, sensory loss, and a permanent loss of utility.
- The exact numbers of compartments in the foot is controversial ranging from 4 to 11:
  - Hind foot—Calcaneal
  - Forefoot—Interosseous (x4) and adductor
  - Full length—Medial, lateral, and superficial
- The loss of pulses or capillary refill is an unreliable sign.
- The loss of two-point discrimination is more reliable than loss of pinprick. Motor loss in trauma patients is very difficult to gauge and should not be used to diagnose compartment syndrome.

Evaluation and Treatment of Ingrown Toenails

Indication

An acutely infected, ingrown toenail is very painful and debilitating. If only one side of the nail plate is involved, a partial nail plate avulsion can be used. However, if the infection is more extensive and involves both sides of the nail plate, then a complete toenail avulsion should be done (Fig. 8-13).

Description of Procedure

- Position the patient supine.
- Local anesthesia should never include epinephrine.
- A toe anesthetic block is usually sufficient. This procedure should not be painful for the patient. If needed, more anesthetic can be added. Often 3 to 5 mL of Marcaine (0.25% or 0.5%) is added to alleviate the postprocedure pain.
- The toe is cleansed in the routine fashion.
- An Esmarch bandage may be used at the ankle or the toe if needed. We do not routinely use them (unless the patient is on aspirin, coumadin, or other blood thinner) because the procedure is brief, and compression of the nail bed usually leads to prompt hemostasis.

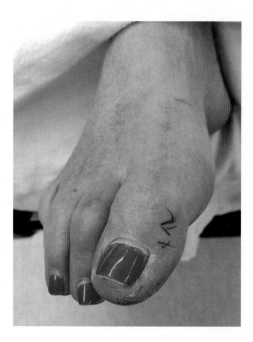

FIGURE
8-13

- The affected, outer edge of the toenail is elevated proximally to the level of the cuticle. A Freer elevator for this part of the procedure is usually used. Make sure to place the freer medial enough (for a medial ingrown toenail) to elevate the ingrown portion of the nail as well. This is accomplished with a sweeping motion (Fig. 8-14).
- Sharp scissors are then used to cut the nail longitudinally for a partial nail plate removal. This step is not needed for a complete toenail avulsion. For a complete avulsion, be sure to use the Freer elevator liberally to elevate the tissues completely medially and laterally (Fig. 8-15).

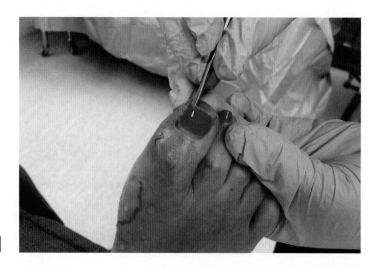

FIGURE
8-14

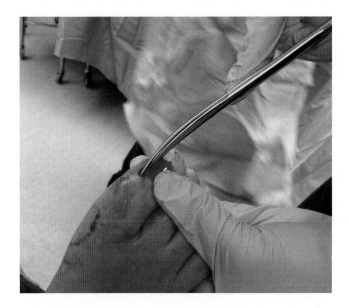

FIGURE
8-15

- A hemostat is used to grasp the nail plate and to avulse it with a rotatory motion, not simply "pulling" the affected nail. This step is especially true for a complete toenail removal. Grasp the nail on one side or the other (not in the center) and rotate the nail to remove. After proper elevation of the nail plate, this step should not be forceful (Fig. 8-16).
- A gauze compression dressing is applied and changed as needed.

Tips and Other Considerations

- Palpate the nail bed after the toenail removal to make sure no spike of nail tissue remains. If so discovered, remove with the hemostat.
- Many patients perceive this to be a painful procedure; allay the patient that the procedure should be relatively painless.

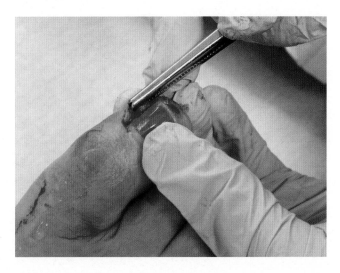

FIGURE
8-16

- After the procedure, educating the patient and "training the tissue" by pushing the ingrown portion of the skin with a cotton-tipped applicator can prevent the ingrown toenail from recurring.
- Although this procedure can give dramatic relief of symptoms, recurrence is high.
- Antibiotics may be prescribed for 5 to 7 days depending on the severity of the infection.

Index

Note: Page numbers followed by *f* indicate figures